INTERPRETIVE
DESCRIPTION

DEVELOPING QUALITATIVE INQUIRY
Series Editor: Janice Morse, University of Utah

Books in the new Developing Qualitative Inquiry series, written by leaders in the field, address important topics in qualitative methods. Targeted to a broad multidisciplinary readership, the books are intended for mid-level/advanced researchers and advanced students. The series will forward the field of qualitative inquiry by describing new methods or developing particular aspects of established methods. Proposals for the series should be sent to the series editor at explore@LCoastPress.com.

VOLUMES IN THIS SERIES

Autoethnography as Method, Heewon Chang

Interpretive Description, Sally Thorne

Developing Grounded Theory, Janice M. Morse, Phyllis Noerager Stern, Juliet M. Corbin, Cathy C. Charmaz, Barbara Bowers, Adele E. Clarke

INTERPRETIVE DESCRIPTION

Sally Thorne

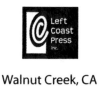

Walnut Creek, CA

Left Coast Press, Inc.
1630 North Main Street, #400
Walnut Creek, California 94596
http://www.lcoastpress.com

Hardback ISBN 978-1-59874-329-6
Paperback ISBN 978-1-59874-330-2

Library of Congress Cataloging-in-Publication Data

Thorne, Sally E. (Sally Elizabeth), 1951-
Interpretive description / Sally Thorne.
p. cm. -- (Developing qualitative inquiry)
Includes bibliographical references.
ISBN 978-1-59874-329-6 (hardback : alk. paper) -- ISBN 978-1-59874-330-2 (pbk. : alk. paper)
1. Education--Research. 2. Education--Research--Methodology. 3. Knowledge management. I. Title.
LB1028.T46 2008
370.72--dc22
2008020775

08 09 10 11 12 5 4 3 2 1

Printed in the United States of America

The paper used in this publication meets the minimum requirements of American National Standard for Information Sciences—Permanence of Paper for Printed Library Materials, ANSI/NISO Z39.48—1992.

Cover design by Andrew Brozyna

CONTENTS

PART II · INTERPRETIVE DESCRIPTION IN PROCESS

PART III · INTERPRETIVE DESCRIPTION IN CONTEXT

FOREWORD

I begin to see that the whole idea of a method for discovering things is ex post facto. *You succeed in doing something, or you do something so well that you yourself want to know how you did it. So you go back, trying to re-create the steps that led you, not quite by accident, not quite by design, to where you wanted to be. You call that re-creation your "method." (Koller, 1983, p. 88)*

This quotation is one of my favorites because it captures what actually happens on the shop floor of research projects, not what is prescribed in instructional research texts. Koller's astute observation also captures a key premise in the book you are about to read. In *Interpretive Description*, Sally Thorne cautions us—researchers both new to and experienced with qualitative research—not to hold to a view of methods that is too methodical. In the "real" world of inquiry, methods are not the fixed entities with unbending rules for implementing them they are depicted as being in the methods literature. In this non-textbook world, things do not happen by planned design, but rather design follows what happens. Departures from textbook renditions of methods are, therefore, not always the violations and mistakes method "purists" lament, but rather reasoned and thoughtful instances of strategic noncompliance. Such noncompliance is strategic (as opposed to misguided) when accomplished by persons who respect the essence and recognize the dynamism of diverse methodological traditions and, thereby, ensure that inquiry will not become stagnant or be held hostage to some putative single right way of doing things. Methods are not procedures to be followed in any standardized way, but rather are created anew in every research project by researchers who hold their work to a standard. Like researchers themselves, methods are dynamic actors subject to historical and cultural change. Novice researchers attempt slavishly to adhere to methods. Seasoned researchers know methodological rules and, thereby, know how to bend them. Some see this as methodological anarchy; others, as methodological innovation.

Thorne's work reminds us that methods are not just ways of gaining access to something heretofore unknown, but also—by virtue of the activities engaged in to secure that access—interventions into or "interference(s)" with the unknown (Mol, 2002, p. 155), and themselves unknowns until efforts are made to use them. *Interpretive Description* reflects Thorne's symbolic interactionist understanding that methods become what they are in the hands of users. Indeed, there is no method apart from a user. When she refers to the "classical" methods of grounded theory, ethnography, and phenomenology, she is not signaling any one ossified entity that exists out there *a priori*, but rather methodological traditions whose histories can be studied and whose current forms reflect changes made in response to scholarly debate and trans-disciplinary trends. Just as the clinical trial we know today did not always exist, or exist in its current form (Gross & Fogg, 2001; Kaptchuk, 1998, 2001), so too have qualitative methods evolved, with, for example, Straussian, Glaserian, neo-positivist, social constructionist, postmodern, and other versions of grounded theory vying for acceptance as the only "true" grounded theory (e.g., Charmaz, 2006; Clarke, 2005; Strauss & Corbin, 1998).

Just as researchers—responding to the varied discourses of postmodernism, postcolonialism, cultural sensitivity, and health disparities, to name a few—are now obliged to fit methods to participants (instead of fitting participants to methods), so too are researchers obliged to fit methods to research purposes. Indeed, Thorne is to be commended for acknowledging and celebrating accommodations of method to the research imperatives and disciplinary agendas of the scholars using them. Interpretive description is such an accommodation, an eclectic but reasoned and mindful integration of theoretical and technical devices to achieve the understandings nurses, physicians, teachers, and other practitioners require to accomplish their respective social missions. As Thorne argues here, methods should never drive research agendas. Researchers should select interpretive description from an array of methodological options when their purposes call for it, and not simply because they want to use it, because they think it easier to use than classical methods, or, like self-described grounded theorists or phenomenologists whose identity derives from these methods, because they want to become "interpretive describers."

Indeed, the most important contribution Thorne makes in this book is in emphasizing the diverse knowledge agendas—visible, in part, in the way methods are used—that separate the practice from other academic/theoretical disciplines. As she suggests here, whereas practitioner/ scholars (e.g., nurses, physicians, social workers, educators, urban planners) see theory as a way to solve real-world problems, academic social scientists see these problems as occasions for theorizing. She and her colleagues (Thorne, Henderson, McPherson, & Pesut, 2004) have warned of the "allure of the binary," but, as binaries go, this is not a bad one as it emphasizes key differences among the disciplines that cannot be ignored. Although social scientists increasingly think of themselves as pursuing intervening disciplines (e.g., Downey & Dumit, 1997), their notion of intervention is hardly the same nor carries the same mandate for improving the public health and welfare as that of the practice disciplines. Accordingly, adaptations of methods cannot be dismissed as simply wrong because they do not comply with *a priori* notions about how a method should be used, but rather understood within a larger trans-disciplinary and social context. Although they often complain about the bastardization of methods in health sciences research, social scientists have much to learn from the health sciences and other practice disciplines about how the methods they claim as their own can be used. As a nurse, I appreciate Thorne's nod to the contributions that nurse researchers and other scholars in the practice disciplines have made to enhance the value and utility of diverse methodological traditions.

No matter what your methodological inclinations or positions, reading this book allows you to have Sally Thorne looking over your shoulder as you conduct your research—to be privy to the insightful and humorous Thornisms that I have enjoyed over the years that she and I have been colleagues and friends and that have shaped my thinking. What a treat for you.

Margarete Sandelowski

Cary C. Boshamer Professor
University of North Carolina at Chapel Hill

REFERENCES

Charmaz, K. (2006). *Constructing grounded theory: A practical guide through qualitative analysis.* London: Sage.

Clarke, A. E. (2005). *Situational analysis: Grounded theory after the postmodern turn.* Thousand Oaks, CA: Sage.

Downey, G. L., & Dumit, J. (Eds.). (1997). *Cyborgs and citadels: Anthropological interventions in emerging sciences and technologies.* Santa Fe, NM: School of American Research Press.

Gross, D., & Fogg, L. (2001). Clinical trials in the 21st century: The case for participant-centered research. *Research in Nursing & Health, 24,* 530–539.

Kaptchuk, T. J. (1998). Intentional ignorance: A history of blind assessment and placebo controls in medicine. *Bulletin of the History of Medicine, 72,* 389–433.

Kaptchuk, T. J. (2001). The double-blind, randomized, placebo-controlled trial: Gold standard or golden calf? *Journal of Clinical Epidemiology, 54,* 541–549.

Koller, A. (1983). *An unknown woman: A journey to self-discovery.* Toronto: Bantam.

Mol, A. (2002). *The body multiple: Ontology in medical practice.* Durham, NC: Duke University Press.

Strauss, A., & Corbin, J. (1998). *Basics of qualitative research: Grounded theory procedures and techniques* (2nd ed.). Thousand Oaks, CA: Sage.

Thorne, S. E., Henderson, A. D., McPherson, G. I., & Pesut, B. K. (2004). The problematic allure of the binary in nursing theoretical discourse. *Nursing Philosophy, 5,* 208–215.

PREFACE

I nterpretive description is a strategy for excavating, illuminating, articulating, and disseminating the kind of knowledge that sits somewhere between fact and conjecture, but which is of central importance to the applied disciplines such as education, community development, human geography, and the health professions. For those whose mandate requires informed action, practicing within the confines of an admittedly imperfect knowledge base is a matter of course. While many elements of our work may be bolstered by conventional science, there is much that has to do with the human experiential and behavioral world of applied practice that requires a distinct form of inquiry. It is this kind of knowledge toward which we turn our attention in this book.

Origins

I have long felt that it is my great good fortune to have found my way into a professional discipline such as nursing. Because it relates to the human experience of health and illness at levels ranging from the cellular to the global, but devotes the vast proportion of its emphasis upon the everyday reality of human-lived experience, nursing indelicately straddles the social and biomedical sciences to find its methodological direction. The kinds of research questions that nurses ask set the stage for the work that they will do to ameliorate human distress, to accommodate bodily frailty, to counter personal vulnerability, and to make meaningful sense of the indignities that life has in store for our bodies and minds. Such questions posed from the framework of a profession so intimately engaged in the mundane and corporeal aspects of health and illness expose those elements of human experience that will permit optimizing the care we provide, better understanding health within its full complexity, and ultimately serving the objects of society for a system of care for those in need. The business of nursing is both vibrant and immediate, having to do with applying patterned knowledge about people in general within the decidedly unique and particular circumstances of the person who sits before you today.

The knowledge that is required in order to advance a profession such as nursing is inherently multifaceted, complex, and diverse. Nurses require reason, philosophy, and science in equal measure, as well as theoretical frameworks with which to synthesize vast bodies of information into a plan of action applicable to an infinite variety of situations. They also need an enormous quantity of practical knowledge to translate the ideas that result from such syntheses into the actual "doing." These features have been a mixed blessing over the discipline's modern history. While nursing's propensity to understand individual experience in context has limited its capacity to advance a more traditional and formal correlational and propositional science, it has also stimulated nurses to seek alternative systematic and rigorous mechanisms by which to uncover understanding and build a knowledge base. It seems, therefore, no accident that nursing has played such a strong leadership role in the evolution of qualitative methods for applied health research over the past generation.

This book reflects one particular development within the application of qualitative research approaches to the specific kinds of problems that the applied disciplines, such as nursing and other health professions, are inclined to raise. Within nursing, the necessity of a research method distinct from the more theoretically driven social science approaches to knowledge development became apparent in the late 1980s, as it grew increasingly evident that attempts to adhere rigorously to the tenets of grounded theory, phenomenology, and ethnography were creating a tension associated with the discipline's requirement for "useable" knowledge. It wasn't that nurses were incapable of understanding or following the rule structures of the methodological traditions they were trying to adopt, but rather that there were subtle yet powerful distinctions between the intellectual projects for which those methods had been created and that of an applied health field. Because qualitative science has been such a "poor cousin" of the more mathematically grounded empirical traditions in health research, inadequately justified adaptations to existing methods were not an option. Rather, a way of thinking through qualitative research logic in relation to a range of distinct kinds of disciplinary questions in a manner that could be both credible and defensible was in order. It was into this context that the approach now called "interpretive description" surfaced.

This book is organized as a guide to both new and more seasoned researchers through the iterative steps of conceiving, designing, and implementing coherent research capable of generating new insights about clinically relevant human phenomena. It illuminates the episte- mological underpinnings and methodological consequences required of a research perspective that will make practical sense and generate credible and useable findings. Drawing thoughtfully upon some of the best analytic maneuvers that phenomenology, ethnography, grounded theory, naturalistic inquiry, and other classic approaches have to offer, it attempts to illustrate how an interpretive description logic model guides researchers through the intricate sequence of study design and implementation to generate research products that hold true to their inherent limitations as well as being meaningful and applicable to dis- ciplinary and professional audiences. In so doing, it articulates a begin- ning-to-end reasoned approach to knowledge development for applied researchers curious about some aspect of human experience within its natural context, and seeking to expand their discipline's capacity to understand the implications of that phenomenon in practice.

How to Use This Book

The design of this book structures ideas in such a manner that it can be used by neophyte qualitative researchers as a "project coach," identify- ing the kinds of challenges and dilemmas that investigators typically encounter at various stages along the way and "talking you through" them. It can also serve as a companion to more seasoned qualitative researchers exploring methodological options, modifications, and re- finements within familiar approaches—a kind of consultation between virtual colleagues such as I have enjoyed with so many of the great authors in the genre. It is therefore written not as a "how to" but rather as an invitation to ask the difficult "how to" questions that inevitably arise in projects addressing clinical problems and to find credible and defensible answers for them.

Graduate students, newer researchers, and established researchers who are attempting to expand their repertoire into the qualitative inquiry domain will find it comforting to have a resource with which to check the logic of their evolving project and that provides some general cred- ibility standards against which to set their methodological reasoning.

Typically, people find their way into interpretive description when the "classic methods" available to them aren't quite fitting the needs of their particular research question. Having reached that insight, they are already well on their way to developing a critical lens in relation to research design choices, and it is that very thoughtfulness this book intends to encourage. Each of the chapters will focus on a distinct element in the conceptualization and implementation of research, but in very few instances will the reader find explicit "how to" direction. Thus, for those seeking a recipe for a quick and easy research project, this will not be the resource of choice. However, researchers wishing to generate methodological options to do justice to the clinical questions that intrigue them will find that the book offers a dialogue in support of rigorous and logical decision making throughout a research project. Within the framework of interpretive description, the chapters will provide guidance toward a product that has both empirical integrity and disciplinary utility.

Since most researchers consult texts at the point of beginning to generate a research proposal, Part One of the book focuses on design decisions and preliminary logic. Part Two speaks to the researcher who is beginning to enter the field, shifting from the grand design to the complicated processes associated with putting that vision into action. Part Three focuses on the intellectual demands of making sense of what one has gleaned and generating credible claims on that basis. As seasoned researchers will know, it is difficult to fully appreciate the demands of each phase of a project until you are in it. Even the most exquisitely articulated research proposal does not really prepare you for the "feel" of the subjective experience of being overwhelmed with data, or losing confidence in your findings. Therefore, this book is envisioned as an ongoing dialogue to guide you as you progress through your research so that you can begin to predict the twists and turns along the way and make effective choices when you come to those inevitable crossroads.

Acknowledgments

In the context of that personal trajectory of coming to an understanding of what it means to hold a methodological logic within the philosophical framework of an applied health discipline, I have been privileged with an extraordinary set of mentors over my career. From my first venture in graduate study, Rose Murakami and Margaret Campbell taught me that thinking as a nurse derives from a fundamental set of philosophical assumptions and positionings that deserve careful attention. Joan Anderson enticed me into the world of qualitative inquiry, recognizing its potential for illuminating some of the intriguing, contextual, and messy aspects that other methods might have stripped away. In a subsequent graduate degree program, Juliene Lipson and Elvi Whittaker brought me further into an appreciation for the pragmatics and politics of method within the social science universe—allowing a standpoint outside of my comfortable disciplinary home. And in subsequent years, my colleague Margarete Sandelowski has ensured that I continue to engage in ongoing intense dialogue about matters of method. If anything I have learned is of worth to others, it is because these intellectual giants have allowed me to engage in and challenge their thinking and push my own understanding at every juncture.

I also owe a sincere debt of gratitude to the many graduate students who have, over the years, engaged with and wrestled with these methodological issues—both my own graduate students and those from other parts of the globe with whom I have corresponded. I have learned so much from your questions and your struggles, and been continually inspired by your aspirations to "do method" in a manner that reflects the integrity of whatever disciplinary logic you bring to your own inquiries. In particular, I'd like to acknowledge the three graduate students (at the time) who participated with me in co-authoring papers on interpretive description as the method evolved: Sheryl Reimer Kirkham, Janet McDonald, and Kathy O'Flynn-Magee and a more recent graduate student, Gladys McPherson, whose insightful reflections on a draft manuscript for this book have enriched it considerably. I have so enjoyed the unfolding of the story of interpretive description through your fine minds.

The qualitative health research community is a rich and diverse one, including a wide range of genuine "characters" and events. Because we have so often had the opportunity for dialogue and engagement at conferences, workshops, and training sessions, we have come to know each other, to push each other's boundaries, and to keep pulling at the underpinnings of what we are doing to see what will happen. From that rich community, I have benefited from many scholarly alliances, and especially wish to acknowledge each of my research partners and co-authors over a long and happy research career. Your fine contributions to my own thinking are well documented in the history of our writing collaborations. And finally, I would like to express a special word of tribute to Jan Morse, whose leadership and persistent optimism that the field of qualitative health research was worth advancing has kept this community dynamic and alive.

Limitations

In a work such as this, the ideas and thoughts that come into the writing derive from years of conversations with oneself and others. Because the world of qualitative study is so incredibly diverse and complex, and because so much has been written about various aspects of it, a commentary such as this one will necessarily do an injustice to the many important ideas that are glossed over, ignored, or oversimplified as part of another argument. Unless this work became a historical study of the rich traditions upon which qualitative health research had been developed, it could not possibly have noted each of the thinkers and writers whose work has informed me over the years. Although some of those greats are acknowledged in formal citation, many equally profound contributors will have been missed in a document whose primary purpose is methodological guidance.

What remains, then, are the thoughts of one individual scholar, presented in the context of a smattering of the relevant background to locate these thoughts within a larger context of evolving ideas, and a good deal of experiential opinion. Where toes are stepped on, contradictory claims left dangling, and half-baked ideas pontificated as if they were fully formed pearls of wisdom, I take full and humble responsibility.

INTERPRETIVE DESCRIPTION
IN THEORY

CHAPTER ONE

Qualitative Research
in the Applied Disciplines

Theorizing and Application

Several years ago I had the experience of engaging in a week-long intensive workshop with a group of academics, composed roughly equally of social scientists and health professional researchers. Although everyone was highly enthusiastic about the topic of discussion (it happened to be genetics and ethics), fundamental schisms began to form quite early in the week between the two groups, such that by the end of the time there seemed an insurmountable impasse. Essentially, for the clinician researchers, the entire point of questing for knowledge was to apply it to real human beings caught in complex and difficult human health problems so that their quality of life could be improved in some manner. For the social scientists, the point of knowledge development was theorizing, and the idea that people would put their ideas to use prematurely was an anathema. While I am well aware that many clinicians theorize and many social scientists do applied work, it seemed that the extreme situation of the workshop had revealed a polarizing tendency that I had not previously appreciated in its fullness. In the context of our interprofessional, multidisciplinary health research world, especially within the qualitative research community, it becomes easy to forget that we do represent distinct disciplines with very different origins and intellectual objectives. After all, we are all friends, working together on projects that are of common interest, and we are all trying to make a better world. We all think of ourselves as enlightened individuals, free thinkers capable of drawing on the ideas and insights of a universe of disciplinary orientations. However, this workshop experience humbled me into grappling with the extent to which we are what we study, and caused me to recognize anew the extent to which the disciplinary traditions into which we are educated shape the angle of vision we take into all of our multidisciplinary activities.

Much of the fine tradition of qualitative health research derives from those social sciences, especially anthropology, sociology, and psychology, from which have evolved such widely known methods as ethnography, grounded theory, and phenomenology (Hamilton, 1994; Vidich & Lyman, 1994). It is therefore important to understand that the intended trajectory of new knowledge in these disciplines is enacted primarily through careful theorizing (Berger & Luckman, 1966; Chenail, 1992; Durrenberger & Thu, 1999; Porter & Ryan, 1996). Anthropology documents and interprets human variations toward enhancing our grasp of what may be universal about being human. Sociology concerns itself with working out the way human nature is manifest in social behavior. And psychology seeks to understand the workings of the human mind, with the social psychology subgroup particularly concerned with the manner in which it plays out in the ways we engage with one another. Although within each of these disciplines there are subspecialists working in an applied "real world" context, the origin of the discipline within human philosophical curiosity ensures that its scholarship remains solidly grounded in theoretical and empirical rather than practical problems (Reason, 1996; Reason & Torbert, 2001; Thorne, 2001).

Applied to the study of health issues, then, the fundamental point of social science research is not to solve everyday problems of patients, but to capitalize on health phenomena to answer problems of a more elemental nature related to understanding how social groups behave and what constitutes the core nature of human experience. To illustrate, there exists a strong sociological tradition of studying epilepsy as a prototypical lens through which to learn more about the workings of social stigma (Goffman, 1968; Scambler & Hopkins, 1990; Schneider & Conrad, 1980). While such work constitutes fine social theorizing and can inform us about the "nonclinical" world in which health and illness are played out, health care professionals and planners would clearly be remiss in assuming this constitutes evidence that epilepsy produces more problematic social disclosure issues than do other chronic diseases.

In direct contrast, applied science within the health disciplines takes its nourishment directly from the clinical context (Chenail, 1992; Miller & Crabtree, 1994). Certainly the applied health disciplines theorize, and often brilliantly so, but when they do, they tend to do so because of a hope that theorizing will produce better application. Essentially, it is in the nature of the clinician to see the human client at the end of the theorizing—to envision the need out there in the world and to want to strive as quickly as possible toward meeting it. In contrast, it is in the nature of the social scientist to see the theorizing as a legitimate and worthy goal in and of itself, and sometimes to see the human being and his or her plight as an opportunity to advance that theorizing. I'm purposefully being extreme here, but I believe that the distinction becomes an important one when it comes to grasping why it is that conventional social science methods cannot advance clinical knowledge in quite the manner that the applied health disciplines require, and why different approaches to discovery are sometimes needed.

The Nursing Example

For those who are not members of the tribe, nursing is a complex and "messy" discipline, having developed on the basis of a common, universal requirement to care for the sick within society and having grown up in partnership with its scientifically oriented cousins in clinical medicine. It has weathered the additional storms of gender bias and economic disadvantage, and has come through a period of political awakening in which it thought of itself primarily as an oppressed group within professional society. It has grappled with what it considers itself—a (quasi-religious) "calling," an occupational group, or a profession—and whether it does or does not possess a distinctive scientific basis apart from medicine and its related health sciences. Further, for much of its modern history, it has attempted to resolve these matters through theorizing, an activity that has often seemed an uncomfortable bedfellow with its practice aims.

However frustratingly problematic the nursing discipline may be, it is also exquisite in its complexity and its purity of purpose. And it is these properties that are important in understanding why nursing's need for knowledge would drive a quest for new methodological options (Dzurek, 1989; Reed, 1995; Sidani, Epstein, & Moritz, 2003; Thompson, 1985; Watson, 1995). Nursing always and inherently requires knowledge about patterns and themes within people in general so that it can better inform the care of the unique and distinct individual. For nursing, knowledge always evolves in dialectic. The care of any individual patient inherently involves examination of the interplay between objective and subjective information, such that technical information about the hip replacement procedure that is about to take place is carefully tempered by the distinctive humanity of the person who is entering that experience. As you discover things about an individual patient, these inform your interpretation and uptake of the available knowledge, which includes not only formal evidence, but also shared clinical wisdom, pattern recognition, established practice, ethical knowledge, and the "how to" of artfully putting all of those together into competent practical application (Johnson & Ratner, 1977; Liaschenko, 1997). You draw upon an amazing array of knowledge sources, sorting and organizing those knowledge options according to a conceptual framework that derives from the philosophical understanding of why we nurse, and on the basis of that organized knowledge you create applications tailored to the specific patient before you today. Even if you are applying a standardized intervention for a health problem you have encountered hundreds or thousands of times before, nursing holds dear the notion that this particular individual may be the one who requires a new twist, a new adaptation, in order to achieve his or her optimal level of health. And this marvelous tension between the general and the particular characterizes the inherent complexity of nursing's intimate relationship with knowledge development.

Of course, nursing's praxis orientation—that dialectic between practice and knowledge—is not unique, and other applied disciplines certainly share many of the same qualities and draw upon many of the same historical thought traditions (Maxwell, 1997). However, nursing is so utterly steeped in them, and they are so central to the core business of the discipline, that forms of knowledge capable of shedding light on that dialectic between conceptualization and action have tremendous value within the everyday practice world. Thus, nursing's comfort within the world of complexity and contradiction, its enthusiasm for ways of thinking that acknowledge the messiness of the everyday practice world, help explain why it would take a lead in what has become a generation of methodological development within the applied qualitative health research field.

Methodological Ancestry

Interpretive description is an approach to knowledge generation that straddles the chasm between objective neutrality and abject theorizing, extending a form of understanding that is of practical importance to the applied disciplines within the context of their distinctive social mandates. It responds to the imperative for informed action within the admittedly imperfect scientific foundation that is the lot of the human sciences.

The methodological form that grew into what is now called interpretive description arose from a need for an applied qualitative research approach that would generate better understandings of complex experiential clinical phenomena within nursing and other professional disciplines concerned with applied health knowledge or questions "from the field." Disentangling methodological strategies from the theoretical assumptions associated with the original social science disciplinary projects for which many of the conventional qualitative research approaches were originally intended, interpretive description reflected the challenge of retaining the coherence and integrity of a theoretically driven approach to knowledge development while supporting defensible design variations according to the specific features of context, situation, and intent. In so doing, it emphasized research design logic as a hallmark of excellent qualitative description of phenomena of concern to the health and applied professional disciplines.

I first wrote about the need for an alternative to the conventional qualitative approaches for applied health research in 1991. At that time, qualitative researchers in the health field were still quite defensive about the quality of their contributions, and tended to rely quite heavily on "established methods" from the social sciences in order to lend credibility to their empirical contributions. Not only did it seem requisite to "locate" oneself within a particular methodological tradition, naming the particular theorists upon whose work one was building, but also one was expected to follow the associated rule structure meticulously (Bartolomé, 1994; Janesick, 1994). However, consideration of the disciplinary projects from which the available methodological traditions derived makes it evident that those rule structures had clear and explicit origins within certain assumptions about knowledge and its creation that were not necessarily applicable (and, at times, in direct contradistinction) to scholarship in the applied context.

As the informed reader will immediately recognize, the disciplines to which I refer and the methodological traditions that have evolved from them over many generations are extensive, complex and multifaceted. They have taken up the working lives of armies of scholars and warranted millions of pages of thoughtful text. In providing a very brief synopsis of each of these fields, I invariably do a great injustice to the integrity of their traditions within the intended context. However, it seems necessary to provide some comment on what these traditions entail before it begins to make sense why I believe that they can't and don't work as *primary* research methods for applied health and professionally motivated knowledge generation.

Ethnography Ethnographic methods as we know them today have evolved over the past century or so as anthropology has attempted to unravel the mysteries of the nature of human existence through careful study of its diverse expressions. Emerging a century ago out of the dominant perspective that "primitive" cultures revealed something of the evolutionary heritage of modern humankind, the ethnographic tradition celebrates human cultural variation as a window into understanding the logic of social organization, cognitive function, and human complexity (Howard & McKim, 1983). It does this through decoding the specific elements of human experience that emerge within the contextual whole of a culture (Sanday, 1983).

In ethnography, direct observation of human behavior and interviewing participants about the meaning of that behavior form central mechanisms for ensuring that the cultural actor's perspective will inform the researcher's analysis. Although scholars have differed on the matter of the extent to which the cultural actor's *emic* view illuminates or blinds us to the more complete *etic* view of a culture (Hammersley & Atkinson, 1983; Kaplan & Manners, 1972; Pelto, 1970; Van Maanen, 1988), most agree that, with the majority of anthropologists themselves the product of a dominant western perspective, a fairly profound degree of relativism has characterized the ethnographic tradition (Hammersley & Atkinson, 1983).

Grounded Theory Grounded theory is an approach whose origins are attributed to the early collaboration between Barney Glaser and Anselm Strauss (Glaser & Strauss, 1967). Reflecting solid sociological origins, its intricate methodological direction derived from the fundamental assumption that human behavior can only be understood within a "collective consciousness" to which the members of the group have no conscious interpretive access (Bowers, 1988; Heller, 1986). Sociology itself arose out of the project of anthropology, with which it was originally closely allied (Strauss, 1987). It departed from the ethnographic enterprise in the extent to which knowledge about the meaning of social behavior is accessible to direct inquiry methods at the local level. Where key informants might provide the anthropologist with the basis upon which to interpret the meaning of certain characteristic behavioral patterns within a society, sociologists felt that the naturalistic and relativistic bias of consciously accessible information was more likely to distract scholars from grasping the underlying network of social structures within which the patterns begin to make larger sense. This distinction between perspectives on whether people's own subjective interpretations of their actions are or are not likely to be accurate in the wider scheme of things is a fundamental feature of the distinct methodological distinctions between grounded theory and its predecessors.

Since the vast majority of sociological activity occurs at the level of understanding the interaction between societies and the individuals who compose them (Outhwaite, 1975; Schwartz & Jacobs, 1979), the objective of sociological research was to understand those social forces that shape human activity (Schatzman & Strauss, 1973). While sociologists might participate in field research in a manner that was somewhat akin to ethnographic study, analysis was firmly located at the dialectic between micro and macro levels (Cicourel, 1981; Fielding & Fielding, 1986). Thus, the products of sociological inquiry using grounded theory are explicitly theory building, in contrast to the ethnographer's pursuit of documenting what sense people make of how they are structuring their world or the phenomenologist's efforts to render articulable those essential elements of subjective human experience that are beyond the reach of normal discourse.

Phenomenology As a methodological derivation of a philosophical stance on fundamental questions of ontology (the nature of being) and epistemology (the nature of knowledge), phenomenology seeks to understand the essential nature of a thing, or those dimensions "without which it would not be what it is" (Van Manen, 1990, p. 10). Phenomenology holds as a central value the premise that the most basic human truths are accessible through the understanding of human subjective experience (Burch, 1989; Cohen, 1987; Giorgi, 1970). Phenomenologists strive to work through the filter of human thinking to obtain knowledge of the deeper essential structure of what it means to be human. "It is the methodology through which I come to understand myself as that ego and life of consciousness in which and through which the entire objective world exists for me, and is precisely as it is" (Husserl, 1929/1975, p.8). As such, within the phenomenological tradition, all knowledge is an interpretation, inevitably made through "exteriorization" of life and reflection upon the effects it produces on others (Ricoeur, 1981b). Phenomenological approaches to research draw on an empathic understanding through sympathetic introspection and reflection—a tradition known as *verstehen* (Patton, 1980). As such, it promotes a fascination for the places of contact between the person and his or her reality (Van Kaam, 1966), especially as brought to expression through linguistic form (Gadamer, 1975/1985; Schutz, 1932/1967). An inherent paradox within phenomenology is that, by generating human consciousness of a truth that is already manifest within the intelligibility of human experience, that truth inevitably changes (Burch, 1989).

Departure and Diversification

In keeping with the disciplinary projects for which they were invented, ethnography, grounded theory and phenomenology spawned complex procedural rules regarding the use and application of their various approaches to inquiry. So, for example, ethnographers developed a set of traditions as to what constitutes fieldwork, and the extent of immersion required in order to make credible claims about a culture. Grounded theory scholars developed rule structures relating to maximal variation of sample, theoretical saturation, and various layers of essential coding. Similarly, phenomenologists developed technique for bracketing prior knowledge, and meticulously distinguishing interpretation from explanation. Because the conclusions a scholar within these disciplines might reach were entirely dependent upon the integrity of the method by which he or she arrived at them, rigid attention to methodological tradition became a primary hallmark of credible qualitative science. While numerous methodological derivations and refinements emerge annually, this adherence to recognizable tradition has remained an important dimension of the scholarly approach to evaluating quality.

When nursing and other health sciences began to take up qualitative methods, this methodological "purity" was generally regarded as essential for rendering qualitative work meaningful within the larger academic health research context. Most of the well-known pioneers in qualitative health research had solid academic grounding within one or another of the traditions, commonly through the socialization of doctoral training. The methodological detail within their written reports made explicit the genealogical heritage they were building upon and many of them became fluent and effective within the theoretical idiom of that discipline.

However, as an increasing number of health researchers began to take up qualitative approaches in an attempt to answer some of the puzzling clinical questions that had not proven amenable to meaningful study using conventional quantitative methods, the limits of the social science approaches when applied to the clinical health context began to surface (Johnson, Long, & White, 2001). While nursing and health researchers had found participant observation and interviewing, the major field methods of ethnography, easily adaptable to the new health-related questions they were posing, they were rarely prepared to examine these clinical phenomena within the larger context of whole cultures (Aamodt, 1989). Instead, they relied heavily upon the formal ethnographies of anthropologists to contextualize their specific findings within a larger understanding of the whole, recognizing that descriptions of specific behaviors, rituals, or beliefs outside of an appreciation for the kinship rules, linguistic patterns, or worldviews of the culture would be dangerously narrow and potentially quite unethical (Germain, 1986; Omery, 1988).

Similarly, while the constant comparative analytic approach derived from grounded theory methodology seemed comfortably similar to the clinical reasoning process with which nurses and other health professionals examine the conditions inherent in each new clinical case against features of all others they have encountered (Chenitz & Swanson, 1986b), rarely were clinicians overly concerned with theorizing the dialectic between social forces and individual interpretation per se. Rather, their analyses tended to acknowledge that social behavior may or may not be at play, and apply that insight to the clinical problem only when it seemed to serve some practical purpose (Hutchinson, 1986; Stern, 1985).

Just as grounded theory and phenomenology differed quite markedly on their positions regarding the use and meaning of subjective knowledge, a similar distinction between the ultimate purpose of phenomenology and the intellectual project of the health disciplines arose in the literature. Because of nursing's historic affinity for application at the level of intimate individual experience, phenomenological methods involving intensive engagement between the knower and the known seemed at face value particularly consistent with the discipline's deeply held moral conviction that each patient represents a unique and deserving individual. Consequently, phenomenology's confirmation of the importance of subjective reality attracted many nursing and health researchers to experiment with its potential for uncovering experiential clinical knowledge (Artinian, 1988; Oiler, 1986). However, in contrast to a more purist phenomenological orientation that sought to uncover the deeper essential structures of "being," and was deeply concerned about assumptions of the extent to which these are or are not shared, the applied health researchers tended to use the method to justify inquiries into those aspects of human health and illness experience that were understood to be sufficiently common as to warrant generalization for the purposes of applying insights to improve sensitive practice (Anderson, 1989). Rather than bracketing the context, they employed it in the selection of topics and emphases, recognizing its dynamic nature in the clinical setting, thereby conflating concern with subjective experience with an analysis of the essential structures underlying it. Thus, in ignoring phenomenology's commitment to the inherent separation of the person from his or her world, applied health researchers attempted to sidestep what have been described as the "incommensurable views on the nature of subjectivity" between the two perspectives (Yegdich, 2000).

While many health scholars unselfconsciously (or perhaps unconsciously) molded and adapted the social science approaches to meet the needs of their qualitative inquiries, others came to recognize that there was an inherent and irreconcilable mismatch. Ethnographers in the anthropological tradition understand human nature as the object of studying variation. Grounded theorists within sociology assume that the value of research is to uncover the tacit basic social processes that drive human action. And phenomenologists within psychology and related fields perceive reality as that which exists because it is experienced through the essential structure of human subjectivity. While each of these disciplinary traditions has a role to play within the larger world of ideas, none of these approaches is compatible with the pragmatic demands of the applied disciplines, whose members find themselves incapable of suspending action until they fully understand a problem (even if they could agree on the nature of that understanding). While they can appreciate the intellectual standpoint that objective and subjective realities may be mutually exclusive, the messiness of everyday practice requires that those within the applied health fields inevitably straddle both. And, therefore, many health researchers found that they had to reject social science methods as the best way to answer qualitatively derived health questions.

With conventional qualitative methodological traditions falling short of the needs of the health research community, a range of explicit and implicit adaptations were beginning to creep into the disciplinary literature. Various researchers blended and borrowed among the available traditions, sometimes making that explicit in their design discussions, but often it was more implicitly evident in their design descriptions, their language choices, and the specific sources from which they acknowledged guidance. Within this context, Janice Morse and others expressed considerable concern that studies maintain a set of standards and avoid sloppiness and "methodological slurring" (Baker, Wuest, & Stern, 1992; Johnson, Long, & White, 2001; Morse, 1989a; Stern, 1994). Other health researchers sought methodological variants from the conventional options, some of which derived from disciplines even further afield from the health project, but perhaps with fewer rules governing their canon. In this context, such alternative approaches as narrative inquiry, autoethnography, ethology, and case analysis started to emerge as descriptors for qualitative health inquiries. This proliferation of claims about research design and method reflected a widespread experimentation toward better ways to legitimize research approaches that would serve the knowledge needs of the disciplines without running afoul of the "methodological police" or detracting from the credibility of the qualitative genre. However, when applied to answering health field questions, many of the products deriving from these diverse approaches still had a similar "look and feel." As Morse observed, there seemed to be a considerable amount of legitimate qualitative research being conducted to address the disciplinary knowledge requirements within the health field for which, to that point, there was "no name" (1989a, p. 6).

The Genesis of Interpretive Description

As had been the case with others within the qualitative health research genre, my own work with excellent colleagues and graduate students increasingly convinced me that it ought to be possible to work out a design logic in alignment with the specific disciplinary requirements for knowledge within nursing and the health professions (Thorne, 1991). I was encouraged in this enterprise by the methodological developments arising from the field of educational studies, in which the particularities of formal methodological adherence had never become such an obsession and whose proponents more easily justified their adaptations by virtue of the decidedly distinct nature of their disciplinary enterprise—having to do primarily with learning rather than being, and with systems rather than individual experiences. In particular, Michael Quinn Patton's contributions to qualitative evaluation research (1987) and the naturalistic inquiry approach advanced by Yvonna Lincoln and Egon Guba (1985) were characterized by a rigorous and thoughtful disciplinary methodology explicitly drawing upon particular elements borrowed from the conventional approaches but reconfiguring them according to the distinctive logic inherent in their new purpose.

Because I recognized that methodological eclecticism was unlikely to produce good science, I became intrigued in my own program of research with the challenge of working out guidelines for qualitative descriptive approaches that would extend beyond mere description and into the domain of the "so what" that drives all applied disciplines. It was apparent that locating clinical research entirely within the theoretical traditions of the social sciences would contribute greatly to social theorizing without necessarily producing knowledge that could be put to any direct applied use. In so many aspects of practice disciplines, there are observable patterns of human behavior or subjective experience that require better understanding, including some "explanatory" interpretive analysis, in order to sort out what aspects require further study, how that might be conducted, and what one might possibly do to work with those patterns in the meantime in the everyday world of practice. This tension between theoretical integrity and utility has come to be quite central to my own thinking, and is the element that drives the overall logic of what we have come to call "interpretive description."

In the mid-1990s, I had the privilege of working with two gradu-ate students who had shown a particular aptitude for wrestling with the integrity of their own design logic, and together we published the original "Interpretive Description" methodological manuscript for a nursing audi-ence (Thorne, Reimer Kirkham, & MacDonald-Emes, 1997). In response to subsequent requests from graduate students and others from diverse applied disciplinary traditions who corresponded with me following the publication of that first paper, we eventually wrote (co-authored with one of the former co-authors and an additional graduate student) a second paper delving further into the analytic process inherent in the method (Thorne, Reimer Kirkham, & O'Flynn-Magee, 2004). These two papers lay out the core of what interpretive description represents conceptually, philosophically, and methodologically, and are the foundation upon which this current book has been constructed. It is a method I have worked with for many years now and have come to believe in; from my experience and that of others, I've developed a solid confidence that it serves a purpose and provides a logic model for generating meaningful scholarly products with application utility in my discipline and the health fields. Others, such as Buissink-Smith and McIntosh in the applied discipline of tourism and leisure studies (1999), have begun to articulate its utility for the develop-ment of knowledge within other applied disciplines beyond the health domain. In writing this book, I "flesh out" the conversation to make more explicit a way of thinking through the unique and particular design chal-lenges that occur in the context of any applied or health study when one tries to blend methodological integrity with a deep understanding of the nature of knowledge within the application context.

What Interpretive Description Is and What It Is Not

By understanding the specific disciplinary origins from which it came and what it hoped to accomplish, the reader can begin to appreciate something of interpretive description's scope and limitations. As will be elaborated in the chapters of this text, interpretive description is not and cannot be a prescriptive, circumscribed sequence of steps that will reliably lead to new discoveries. Neither is it an entirely novel or distinctive approach, proposing methodological options that would not be familiar to those who work within the more established qualitative approaches. Nor is it qualitative description stripped entirely of its theoretical or disciplinary underpinnings, an approach that also plays a useful role in the development of new knowledge (Sandelowski, 2000).

Rather, I see it as a way of naming and referencing the kind of well-founded logic that clinical researchers have been coming up with in many of what I would consider the most highly respected applications of qualitative research within the health domain. Providing a name and a *raison d'être* for interpretive description as presented here is a more appropriate and viable option than watering down or modifying phenomenology, ethnography or grounded theory and hoping no one notices the methodological violations (Johnson, Long, & White, 2001), or simply calling it "qualitative description" (Sandelowski, 2000) or considering it "generic qualitative research" (Caelli, Ray, & Mill, 2003) stripped of explicit quality criteria. Interpretive description becomes a conceptual maneuver whereby a solid and substantive logic derived from the disciplinary orientation justifies the application of specific techniques and procedures outside of their conventional context. By allowing us to organize around a disciplinary conceptual frame, it permits us to build up a body of knowledge about the implications of design options in relation to the infinite universe of clinical phenomena that we might reasonably wish to know more about, and it provides us with a solid and defensible basis upon which to judge whether a particular piece of qualitative output is worthy of our serious attention.

Interpretive description is a qualitative research approach that requires an integrity of purpose deriving from two sources: (1) an actual practice goal, and (2) an understanding of what we do and don't know on the basis of the available empirical evidence (from all sources). It constitutes a method that generates questions from that grounding, pushes one into the "field" in a logical, systematic and defensible manner, and creates the context in which engagement with the data extends the interpretive mind beyond the self-evident—including both the assumed knowledge and what has already been established—to see what else might be there. As such, it offers the potential to deconstruct the angle of vision upon which prior knowledge has been erected and to generate new insights that shape new inquiries as well as applications of "evidence" to practice. While, like all qualitative research, its claims to generalization and evidence-generation must be understood as tenuous, the evidence-based practice context in which health decisions are being made on a daily basis makes it increasingly important that we have access to methods that allow us to critically interpret why the current state of empirical science is the way that it is and what that might mean. We desperately need new knowledge pertaining to the subjective, experiential, tacit, and patterned aspects of human health experience—not so that we can advance theorizing, but so that we have sufficient contextual understanding to guide future decisions that will apply evidence to the lives of real people.

As the reader will discover, the treatise on interpretive description that this book represents will fail as a "cookbook" in that there will be very few guidelines that are prescriptive and explicit. It will provide much more substantive understanding of what to avoid than what one must do to ensure the integrity of a project, since various design elements become either brilliant or ludicrous depending on the research context to which they are applied. Rather, what it will do is invite the reader into a conversation about the meaning and nature of the disciplinary project on behalf of which he or she wishes to ask research questions, and to encourage qualitative design decisions in keeping with the nature of the discipline and its question. It will attempt to model a design logic that has an integrity for acceptable science and to the philosophical underpinnings of the applied disciplinary world—in essence, to help the reader grapple intelligently with the "how to" in conjunction with the "why."

Cultivating Questions
in the Clinical Field

What's the Question?

Research questions don't simply materialize out of thin air. In the context of such disciplines as those within applied health, they very clearly derive from the universe of clinical problems for which the available knowledge is not yet sufficient. Beyond their contextual origins in the clinical setting, research questions also have explicit derivation within the academic "project" of various disciplines—in other words, they require a grounding within a reason for inquiry before the specific new question makes any sense. This disciplinary orientation is what distinguishes a research question from one that is merely journalistic or curiosity-driven. Indeed anyone can gather data and make claims (as the internet explosion so powerfully illustrates), but only those who have credibly located themselves within the scholarship of a discipline and/or the mandate of a *profession* can legitimately generate qualitative findings that have meaning as empirical disciplinary knowledge.

Although it may seem self-evident that research quality depends upon the match between the question and the method, the act of generating questions is itself a complex mental operation. Here we examine some of the inherent challenges in the process and invite reflection on the nature of questions in general before entering into a discussion on how one might frame questions within the interpretive description context.

Where Have We Come From?

In conventional (quantitative) health science, the grounding of new inquiry upon existing knowledge is well understood; it becomes a significant component of what distinguishes a worthy scientific claim from a data-referenced "spin." But qualitative research within the health fields has at times followed a different path, perhaps because of its distinct history and tradition within the larger context of health research. I trace the enthusiasm for qualitative health research to the seminal contributions of social science giants such as Goffman (1961), Sudnow (1967), Strauss (1975), and Kleinman (1980). Inspired by such work, by the middle of the 1980s, a cadre of pioneering nurse researchers, such as Anderson (1981), Field and Morse (1985), Leininger (1985), Parse and colleagues (1985), Chenitz and Swanson (1986a), and Munhall and Oiler (1986) had begun to advocate for the adoption of this new "paradigm" of scientific progress in which the inherent complexities of human subjectivity and social behavior could become a central focus of inquiry instead of simply a contaminant within the research process.

These early qualitative health research proponents typically adopted a Kuhnian (Kuhn, 1962) paradigmatic stance to the understanding of "scientific revolutions," and for at least a decade located qualitative efforts as explicitly contrary to the logical positivism from which quantitative approaches were presumed to derive. Thankfully, our community of scholarship has evolved on the basis of a deeper understanding of the philosophical perspectives shaping our epistemological and ontological disciplinary stances. However, for a time, the world of health research seemed quite polarized into the two kinds of research, as if they were inherently mutually incompatible and their proponents were incapable of even understanding shared research problems, let alone working together to resolve them. This history may help explain some of the defensiveness that can be detected in earlier qualitative work (and that still creeps into some contemporary reports) and some of the choices that were made by various scholars in framing and presenting their work.

What Constitutes a Qualitative Question?

Qualitative research typically seeks to generate empirical knowledge about human phenomena for which depth and contextual understanding would be useful, and for which measurement is inappropriate or premature. While quantitative science has generated marvelous traditions within which information about groups and populations can be distilled, qualitative scholars tend to focus upon patterns and themes within individual human experience. To some extent, they reflect distinctions between objective and subjective knowledge, between confirming value-neutral truths and depicting experiential reality.

Understanding the difference between the general epistemological stances from within which the methodological traditions derive is important because it ensures that you align the methods by which you seek answers with the nature of the questions you are asking in the first place. You can't draw conclusions about how people "feel" from documenting how they "behave"; nor can you sum up people's perceptions of a situation and conclude that unanimity confirms that you have a generalizable "truth." Sometimes it is difficult distilling the specific question that might be amenable to research out of a complex set of clinical issues that intrigue you. And in that context, an important step of the research process involves clarifying the various options you have for distilling out a researchable problem and posing it in such a manner that it can draw upon formal research method for an answer.

For example, if you were interested in providing better care for patients in chronic pain, you might consider evaluating the equivalence of various pain measures, experimenting with different protocols for enhancing intervention, or exploring the worldview of those who had lived long enough with the phenomenon to form opinions about how various care options were subjectively received. Each is a worthy objective, and each requires an entirely different research approach. On the basis of each of these, you might be able to generate a study that yielded some answers, but only about the question you had posed. So, for example, by comparing pain measures, you might indirectly help enhance the work of those who intervene or give care, but you could not claim conclusions about those elements directly.

When we understand the nature of a qualitative question, we can think through what it is and what it is not and, using our logic, predetermine appropriate methods by which it might be tackled and the scope and limits of what we might be fortunate enough to find. Being able to think through the relationship between a problem, a question, a method and the eventual research product is an essential skill in becoming proficient in research. If this is your first attempt, you may find it very challenging to think more than one or two steps ahead of yourself, and for this reason, most of us require experienced guides to take us on our first such journey. In the absence of such guidance, you might consider creating a research "support team" (often other neophyte researchers are equally eager to connect and share ideas) or generating a virtual dialogue. While seasoned scholars often become quite comfortable in solo qualitative research, the majority of us learn the tradition best with a combination of intensive reading, reflecting, conversing, and wrestling with ideas. Because, despite great advances in software and technology, qualitative research relies completely on the mental agility of the researcher, drawing upon a variety of strategies to get your mind in shape for the challenge is strongly recommended.

What Constitutes a Disciplinary Question?

Beyond serving as a convenient mechanism for dividing up buildings within universities, academic disciplines play an important role in creating communities of scholars who can build upon a common set of foundational building blocks to drive knowledge development in particular directions. While an academic department will typically house a wide range of scholars working on quite different elements of disciplinary knowledge, the underlying structure, assumptive set and intentionality of their academic discipline will create a coherence that allows them to, for example, build curriculum, decide whether a thesis is or is not acceptable, and bring their various scholarly projects into an understanding of a coherent whole. That may seem to oversimplify the current status of academic disciplines that have become marvelously diverse and complex, but I think it remains an important piece of the puzzle in understanding why, in our interdisciplinary world, disciplines continue to play an important role.

In the medical science context, we are comfortably familiar with the value of explicitly capitalizing upon different orientations toward a problem. Where a medical emergency involves multiple organ systems, the competing perspectives of relevant medical subspecialists will ensure that the rights of each organ are considered in the development of solutions. In this context, we appreciate that each angle of vision "advocates" for a particular perspective, and we generate dialogue among those perspectives to create what are understood to be the best solutions. At the same time, we fully appreciate that it is the "whole person" who stands to lose if the decision is wrong, and we trust each of those subspecialists to critically weigh the conclusions derived from his or her specialty perspective against the whole situation. Thus, we appreciate the value that diversified interests and perspectives bring to a problem, and we would not tend to want to homogenize them into a lesser degree of knowledge about many specialties held by a single practitioner.

In the interdisciplinary academic context, the same principle applies, although many scholars seem to have forgotten this in their enthusiasm to embrace a spirit of cooperation and collaboration. In an earlier era in which interdisciplinary study was often considered inherently weak and unprincipled, we had problems deriving from the inability to collaborate and share (much like what would occur in the fragmented context of medical decision making if the subspecialists refused to engage in respectful dialogue). Because of that, much of the current interdisciplinary fervor seems a reaction to that earlier divisiveness. We comfortably study together, borrow knowledge, appropriate methods, and (at times) seem to be speaking the same language. However, while that new spirit of cooperation fosters some excellent new partnerships, it can also create a climate within which people pick and choose ideas without understanding their heritage and context, and unwittingly generate intellectual claims that are impossible to evaluate, judge, or contest.

Some examples from my own discipline may illustrate this point. Nursing is a professional discipline explicitly mandated to apply knowledge to the resolution of human health and illness problems within society. While it may sometimes be difficult to explicitly delineate the boundaries of that disciplinary orientation, that doesn't mean they don't exist. Early in my career, the common disciplinary wisdom was that violence against women was not a problem of specific concern to nurses, and was more properly the domain of social workers and the judicial/correctional systems. Fortunately, many nurses pushed that boundary in their scholarship and application, and the relevance of violence today as a health problem deserving of nursing attention would not be in question. However, simply because a disciplinary boundary can expand with new knowledge does not imply that it should be erased. Should nursing therefore justify involvement within any aspect of knowledge development that might conceivably involve people, since they have the potential to become ill? Or are there aspects of the study of violence that are more properly the domain of psychology, criminology, or policing? A classic example of the discipline invoking its boundary occurred several years ago when a respected scholarly nursing journal published a research report on career-oriented women with tattoos (Armstrong, 1991). While a report pertaining to that topic might have been of some interest to various disciplines (within sociology, as an instance of new behavior trends; within psychology, as an instance of peer pressure or poor impulse control; within public health, as a potential infection vector), this particular paper described the phenomenon in a nonproblematic manner, such that nurses could not detect any link to clinical application potential. In subsequent letters to the editor, readers angrily charged the journal with abandoning relevance as a quality criterion.

This idea of disciplinary relevance crosses all disciplinary boundaries. As humans blessed with the gift of infinite curiosity, all academics are capable of being intrigued about ideas that are not central (or even marginally related) to their disciplines. Sometimes the insights derived from "being in the world" in this manner do actually inform and enrich our disciplinary scholarship. However, abandonment of "the discipline" slides us into the fuzzy world of knowledge for knowledge's sake.

Detached from our disciplinary histories and allegiances, we begin to lose our grip on the capacity to distinguish good and bad science, right and wrong ideas. Because of this, the orthopedic surgeon who develops a fascination for adolescent linguistic patterns because his or her teenagers have started to use foul language is no more a credible scientist within that field than would be the local police officer. Our understanding of the distinct nature of a scientific claim derives at least as much from the disciplinary source as it does from the relative truth or falsehood of the conclusion—even though very good ideas may sometimes arise from those without formal grounding in a field precisely because they aren't blinded by its assumptions. Thus we understand that the nature of a claim, and the expectations of how it might legitimately be taken up in society, is contingent on the foundations upon which it was made.

In my opinion, this stricture applies not only to topic, but also to method, and in the current context to the kinds of methods that one will choose in order to do credible and valuable research. I have made a case that applying disciplinary methods outside of the disciplinary project for which they were intended tends to create problems—either with the integrity of the methodological application or with the eventual relevance of the results. Similarly, selecting the research questions one will ask simply on the basis of a fascination for a particular method seems to have missed the point. As my colleague Margarete Sandelowski often puts it, we don't want to teach people to *be* grounded theorists or phenomenologists; rather we must teach them to apply the methods that are appropriate to the answering of real and meaningful research questions within their fields. So, for example, I see a significant difference between working with the thematic analysis elements of grounded theory methodology to discern patterns within the shared experience of persons with a similar health challenge and using narrative analysis to deconstruct the structural elements of someone's illness story. What we learn using one method provides us with an appreciation for pattern; what we learn from another gives us insight into how people engage in "the telling." The point is that, because different approaches will lead to different kinds of knowledge, our methodological selection ought to derive from what it is that we are looking for.

What's Worth Studying Qualitatively?

The kinds of disciplinary problems or questions for which one might turn to interpretive description are those for which there is some justifiable rationale for generating or expanding upon existing descriptive knowledge. While one might argue that anything that interests us is worth describing, that seems a rather hollow justification for expenditure of empirical energy, and perhaps a co-option of science toward selfish ends. The better rationale comes from an understanding of how careful and rigorous description, expanding or extending upon what is already "known," would enhance our ability to engage with a particular phenomenon of some clinical interest. I am therefore quite serious about the notion that individual curiosity, on its own, is quite insufficient to justify a scientific project within a practice discipline.

At the outset of a study it is wise to reflect on what constitutes a valid topic. Readers may well have noticed that, within the health literature for example, there are numerous reports of qualitative studies that seem to have been generated for all the wrong reasons. It seems unjustifiable, for example, to generate a new qualitative study simply because one is unwilling to read what has already been written on the topic. Further, it is hard to defend a claim that new investigation is required simply because one's own distinct client population was not included in prior investigations or because the methodological approach differed from that which is now proposed. It seems even less justifiable to launch a formal study into a topic that has attracted your attention simply because it affects you personally; indeed, the fine line between autoethnography and personal therapeutic work is one that I think demands very careful and thoughtful delineation and "location" within the existing body of knowledge. After all, as proponents of science, we qualitative researchers have a privileged position within the world of ideas. If the products of our inquiries are to have empirical advantage in comparison to the products of opinion, persuasion, or even fiction, it behooves us to ensure that our arguments for the value of each new study within the larger context of an evolving body of accessible knowledge are solid, coherent, and reasonable.

Although, in an earlier era, scholars tended to think that the distinct worldviews of qualitative and quantitative research were sufficiently mutually exclusive to preclude their coexistence, researchers in many fields—including health and other applied disciplines—have long since recognized that complex topics demand the application of multiple methods so that we can move beyond advancing method and toward advancing substantive understanding (Miller & Crabtree, 1999a). While this cross-method capacity may occur in collaborative teams, each member bringing his or her own methodological expertise to the table, it increasingly can be found in the repertoire available to creative researchers. Consequently, the ability to discern and detect the kinds of problems and knowledge development trajectories for which a qualitative method will be the most meaningful option has become important and relevant to the discussion.

It is rare that a qualitative study can be justified with the claim that "nothing is known" about the topic. Very likely, quite a lot will be known, but perhaps not within the intellectual circles to which the author is making reference. That which is worth studying qualitatively is credibly argued when the next logical question in advancing disciplinary knowledge is one for which themes and patterns have not been well documented, for which the subjective or experiential elements of the phenomenon are not yet fully reported, or for which the links between known elements and the larger experiential context have not been effectively made. And for good measure, what is worth studying is that which may have some relevance and utility to the mandate that has been granted to the discipline by the society that supports it.

Generating Questions in Interpretive Description

Having considered the matter of what constitutes a qualitative research question and the intellectual heritage upon which such questions can be built, we turn specifically to the topic of how to extract direction for identifying, articulating, and framing research questions that will be consistent with the disciplinary objects and methodological possibilities offered by interpretive description.

Finding a Researchable Problem

In my experience, thoughtful clinicians generally have little difficulty generating lists of clinical curiosities and practice problems that might prove amenable to formal inquiry. However, in the typical situation, these tend to be initially articulated as very loose and preliminary formulations for ideas that could potentially lead into researchable questions, but not without some considerable effort. While curiosity-driven inquiry has its place within the scheme of human learning, the process of moving general inquisitiveness into the scientific formulation of a researchable problem takes us into the literature (both scientific and otherwise) to see what established scholars consider known and not known about this and related concepts or ideas.

Fortunately, a formal critical literature review by a thoughtful inquirer does sharpen one's grasp of the larger field and what can be said about it. Reading what others have written typically gets you increasingly excited about the value of knowledge and much wiser about the value of the various options for developing it. With the rapid proliferation of accessible knowledge, it is incumbent upon the researcher to demonstrate a logic trail through which decisions pertaining to background resources have been constructed. Thus, you don't get to claim that something constitutes a researchable problem until you have done your homework to build the case that it isn't already known and that it is, in fact, worth knowing. Because this obligation is a hallmark of all formal research, this immersion into the ideas of others becomes an inherent part of the process of formulating a good research problem on the basis of what began as simply wondering about a clinical matter. We'll say more about the literature review process in the next chapter.

Framing a Research Question

The syntactic form that transforms the researchable problem into a research question is of critical importance, since it will shape your entire process and influence the degree to which your research project meets with success in achieving its objectives. I would recommend that careful attention be put to this stage, and that the final form of both the problem statement and the formal question be suspended until a wide range of options have been considered.

An example might best illustrate the complexity involved in writing what often ends up in the form of a simple sentence. If you had determined that it was justifiable and important to extend our current understanding of how some persons with disabling conditions become models of health promotion, you might experiment with the conceptual labels to which you were anchoring your question, considering, for example, the implications of choosing terminology to describe the population (such as "handicapped," "chronically ill," or "mobility-challenged") and the descriptor (such as "wellness," "optimal health," or "quality of life"). By reviewing recent writings or attending professional meetings on the topic, you might familiarize yourself with the political, disciplinary, or ideological implications associated with the various choices, and select terminological options that will most effectively communicate what you think you are doing and for whom.

You might then work on the various options for linking those concepts within the grammatical form of the actual question, experimenting with strong associations (correlation? cause?) or softer ones (association? relationship?). Further, you might play with considerations of what the question looks like if grounded in different interrogative sentence forms. These can begin with a question (such as "what," "how," or "when") or an auxiliary verb (such as "would," "can" or "do"). Since many of us become fixated upon certain initial framings of our ideas (sometimes the words that first came to us when we became conscious of our interest in the idea, or a neat turn of phrase that we have heard or read in relation to the topic), it can be very helpful to solicit the input of others at this stage, as their minds may offer alternative formulations we hadn't thought of. For most of us, this intellectual sharing takes its initial form in the graduate seminar, and with any luck continues with valued colleagues and students throughout a research career.

From this process, you should be able to generate a selection of good options for consideration before selecting the ideal question. From the above example, one can see that there will be profound differences between such options as "How do mobility-challenged persons define wellness?" and "What strategies and resources do highly functioning persons with disability identify as being most conducive to a positive quality of life?" An experienced researcher will be able to rapidly project the mind forward from each of these questions to identify what it would imply for all phases of the research process and for the eventual product. For the neophyte, it will be important to reflect on what the question implies as far as such matters as, Who would I be studying in order to learn this? What would I have to find out from them in order to begin to answer this question? How would I gather that kind of data? What categories or groupings of information does my question imply I am seeking? What would it matter if I were able to answer this question?

Typically, a reflective process such as this accomplishes two valuable ends. First, it does help you nail down a question that is sufficiently well articulated to sustain a logical and coherent (not to mention manageable) research project. Second, it opens up your awareness to the actual scope and boundaries of the question you have posed—what it is and what it is not. Since many of us enter clinical research with multiple questions, it can be painful to "let go" of some of the many additional hidden agendas we have when we enter a study. However, if we don't, we run the risk of confusing agenda with interpretation. The power of a good question—and of truly understanding the nature of the question you have posed—is that it keeps your logic focused when the complexity of the field makes the analytic process most confusing. And this capacity to maintain a clarity of purpose is what will ensure

TEXT BOX 2.1

Chemotherapy-Induced Peripheral Neuropathy

Bakitas used an approach informed by interpretive description to study how patients live and cope with experiencing the symptoms of neurotoxicities associated with commonly used cancer therapies. The findings metaphorically represented these unpleasant sensory, motor, and autonomic symptoms as "background noise" influencing everyday life for these individuals. Patient descriptions of how they became aware of these symptoms, came to understand them, and learned how to deal with them vividly illuminate the pervasive disruption these symptoms signify in daily life. They further document the amazing capacity of people living with cancer to adapt to the adverse effects of this disease.

Bakitas, M. A., (2007). Background noise: The experience of chemotherapy-induced peripheral neuropathy. *Nursing Research, 56*(5), 323–331.

that the final conclusions are credibly grounded in the empirical data that you produce. So although it may seem silly, the value of really generating the right research question cannot be underestimated.

Clarifying Questions Amenable to Interpretive Description

A somewhat facetious way of explaining which kinds of questions are amenable to interpretive description is that it is best suited to those questions that beg an inductively derived description of a phenomenon, and one that deserves an interpretive lens. However, what that means cannot be fully appreciated until we consider a somewhat more refined answer to the questions: What is description? And what is interpretation?

What Is Description? In the research sense, the term "description" is used to explain studies whose purpose is itemizing or documenting something that requires it—telling what it is that one observed (Sandelowski, 2000). The term explicitly differentiates this kind of inquiry from that which seeks to test a theory or prove a relationship, and merely reports to us, using a set of inquiry conventions compatible with the intent, what can be seen when one examines a phenomenon. Qualitative description is typically understood to differ from that which is quantitative in terms of its degree of reliance on objective (especially numeric) data as opposed to those that are only accessible through human subjectivity. However, this is something of a false dichotomy, and it may sometimes be more useful to draw the distinctions between the form of logic (deductive or inductive) upon which the method relies. Qualitative description builds findings based on inductive reasoning, while quantitative description builds them by deducing. Deductive reasoning moves from the more general toward the specific, so that one might begin with a theory and use descriptive techniques to confirm its applicability within a particular specific instance. Inductive reasoning works the other way, building from specific observations of a thing toward broader generalizations or theories. By its very nature, then, qualitative description will be open and exploratory, in contrast to the more narrow and focused description that would be sought using quantitative techniques.

According to Sandelowski (2000), descriptive research has often been depicted as the least impressive or valuable form of both quantitative and qualitative research. Perhaps because of the quantitative tradition in which strong findings require experimental approaches, qualitative researchers in the health field have been reluctant to depict their work as "mere" description. Rather, they have often portrayed their work as phenomenology, grounded theory, narrative, or ethnography in order to ascribe to it some "epistemological credibility" (Thorne, Reimer Kirkham & MacDonald-Eames 1997), or what Woolcott has depicted as methodological "posturing" (1992). Like Sandelowski, in advancing interpretive description as a methodological option, I am hoping to revitalize an enthusiasm for description as a powerful resource in the knowledge development armament. While our approaches differ on the relevance of disciplinary grounding to a good "qualitative description," we are both working toward a better level of intellectual honesty and methodological integrity in the scholarly products that are generated within our traditions. For the health field, description is and will remain an extremely important element in bringing phenomena to the awareness of our colleagues, in creating an empirical basis from which new questions can be generated, and for taking note of the manifestations of the complex and messy world of human health and illness.

What Is Interpretation? When we add the descriptor "interpretive," we are explicitly locating our studies of human social phenomena within a nondualistic philosophical tradition (Crotty, 1998). In so doing, we distinguish our work from dualistic research approaches derived from assuming the rational and empirical aspects of the mind are in inherent opposition to one another. Instead, we draw inspiration from philosophical underpinnings that explicitly capitalize on the perspective that reality doesn't exist "out there" as an objective entity to be discovered but rather is more usefully understood as "socially constructed" through the subjective person who experiences it (Mottier, 2005). This "interpretive turn" grew out of a tradition generated by such thinkers as Paul Ricoeur (1981a), Martin Heidegger (1982), and Hans-Georg Gadamer (1989), which focused attention upon the analysis of construction of meaning within subjective and intersubjective experience. Research drawing on these ideas involves cultivating the skill of appreciating experience from the perspective of others, while simultaneously accounting for the cultural and social forces that may have shaped that perspective. Because the point of such research is not simply to interpret action through the motivations that are accessible to subjective consciousness, but to concentrate on the lived context within which those actions evolve and become meaningful, inquiry involves a dialectic that has come to be known as the "hermeneutic circle."

Although many qualitative health researchers have drawn heavily on the insights of these authors (as they do on the excellent work of the full range of social science methodologists), it remains important to remember that these approaches to inquiry were developed to address the very specific intellectual challenges that were at the forefront of thinking of particular disciplinary groups at specific points in time. Because of this, full adherence to the methodological requirements of many of these foundational sources draws one into a different sort of conversation, and sometimes away from the one that generated the health research question in the first place. So, for example, although an appreciation for the dialectic between power and oppression can be an exciting focus of intellectual curiosity, it may be more suitable for developing grand theorizing than for trying to resolve the day-to-day problems of marginalized members of society. Thus the "interpretation" that has evolved within the qualitative health field, while informed and excited by these marvelous alternative "standpoints" from which to examine problems, still relies upon the more practical, analytical "so what might this mean?" form of interpretation that extends description beyond documentation and into sense-making (Benner, 1994). Norman Denzin has elaborated an action research method, "interpretive interactionism," as an explicit approach to interrogating the interrelationship between what he calls "private lives and public responses to personal troubles" (1989, p. 10). His approach begins and ends with the biography of the researcher, and generates thick description and epiphanies that contribute to a better understanding of how we socially construct power, knowledge, history and emotion (p. 19). Since this technique capitalizes on "auto-reflection" (to use Denzin's term) and theoretical deconstruction, it too is limited in the utility it will have as the guide to methodology for the majority of applied qualitative inquiries.

What Is Interpretive Description? What the interpretive description approach considers "interpretation," then, takes inspiration from the formal interpretive hermeneutic tradition without becoming a confirmed believer. It recognizes that the clinical mind tends not to be satisfied with "pure" description, but rather seeks to discover associations, relationships and patterns within the phenomenon that has been described. When we qualitatively describe a clinical case, for example, we do so not simply for the documentary value of having recorded it, but because of the inherent assumption that there may be other cases out there that bear some relevant similarity, and that by making this one accessible, we move one step closer to general knowledge. We therefore inherently work within the world of studying instances and integrating what we learn about them with our reflective clinical reasoning process, searching for underlying meanings that might further illuminate what is happening and develop a deeper appreciation toward what would ultimately be the optimal clinical response (Crabtree & Miller, 1999a).

In this way, interpretive description reflects a kind of mental attitude that is consistent with a significant proportion of the clinical questions that might be amenable to qualitative description filtered within a disciplinary lens. It suggests that there is inherent value in careful and systematic analysis of a phenomenon and an equally pressing need for putting that analysis back into the context of the practice field, with all of its inherent social, political, and ideological complexities. Thus it challenges the scholar to be looking below the self-evident within a clinical issue—to be documenting patterns and themes among examples of a thing, and to reconfigure what is found into a form that has the potential to shift the angle of vision with which one customarily considers that phenomenon.

To achieve this aim, interpretive description research questions should ideally be articulated in such a manner that they extend our reach beyond generic qualitative description (typically reflected in such questions as, What is happening here? What are the dimensions of the concept? What variations exist?) and into the domain of interpretive explanation (How are phenomena similar or different from one

---

TEXT BOX 2.2

The Context of Cultural Sensitivity

Reimer Kirkham used interpretive description to study the experiences of recently graduated registered nurses with caring for patients from different cultures. In the context of an increasingly diverse population base, Reimer Kirkham wanted to better understand what it is like for these new nurses to confront the challenges associated with diversity and the extent to which their educational programs had prepared them for this aspect of professional practice. What this researcher found was that caring for clients whose cultural background was different from their own was both challenging and rewarding, and that nurses ranged in their attitudes on a continuum from resentful to embracing diversity. As the nurses described their creative approaches to the complex challenges, Reimer Kirkham was able to extract and interpret common patterns in their views about the conditions under which the skills of cultural competence were supported or discouraged within the clinical practice context. The findings of this study help us better understand the dynamics of culturally insensitive care as well as offering strategic direction toward realizing the goal of a more sensitive and effective system.

Reimer Kirkham, S. (1998). Nurses' descriptions of caring for culturally diverse clients. *Clinical Nursing Research, 7*(2), 125–146.

---

another? How to they relate to one another? What patterns exist? And how do they operate?). Of necessity, interpretive description questions must stop short of formal explanatory pretensions (causation, prediction, control, evaluation), for these become the domain of a much different form of inquiry.

Achieving the alignment between a question and the methodological tools with which it will be answered is the most fundamental of research skills and, unfortunately, the one with which so many qualitative researchers have encountered difficulty. Using interpretive description, which is designed to mimic the interpretive mental attitude that is the hallmark of applied health clinical reasoning processes, and guiding that perspective within the formal methodological traditions for sampling, data collection, and data analysis generated on behalf of descriptive qualitative inquiry, the researcher is invited to work within pressing problems of his or her own disciplinary field and to generate credible and defensible new knowledge in a form that will be meaningful and relevant to the applied practice context.

CHAPTER THREE

Scaffolding a Study

Scaffolding a study sets up the initial position from which you will build out your design plan. Decisions you make in this stage can have a significant impact throughout the project. The scaffolding process feels something like preparing the ground upon which you want to put up a tent for the night. First, you need to survey the broad options— should you position it on high ground or low, near trees or out in the open? You may have some fundamental requirements (relatively flat, near the campfire) and some less pressing but still important considerations (angle of sunrise, proximity to neighbors). Taking all of these into consideration, you decide on the general spot and then survey it for the specific implications of how it will position your tent floor (Are there rocks that you can't relocate? Knobby tree roots in the way? Swarms of nesting insects in that particular spot?). What you discover may lead you to rethink your initial location decision. Having determined the specific spot, you will want to comb the ground for sharp stones that may puncture your sleeping mattress, or cover it with soft grasses to buffer natural bumps in the terrain. You will also want to trench the perimeter of the tent floor space to encourage an appropriate flow of drainage. Only then are you prepared to put up the tent, ensuring that each peg is in its proper place and each rope is appropriately taut. This exercise becomes natural to seasoned campers because they fully appreciate the implications of failure to go through each step in sequence. When the deluge of rain comes, as it inevitably will one night, the carefulness of this preparation will distinguish the camper in the soggy sleeping bag from the one who has a dry and enjoyable camping experience.

To find your way safely through the predictable hazards of an interpretive description research project, you have to know who you are, what you represent, and what you are trying to accomplish. In essence, you need to sort out what intellectual positioning you are taking into the project; what assumptions, values, and beliefs they represent; what "facts" you are considering as known and not known in relation to the topic; and what it is that you'll be seeking to find. In our early writings on interpretive description, we used the language of "analytic framework" (Thorne, Reimer Kirkham & MacDonald-Eames, 1997) to refer to the background knowledge and disciplinary orientation that one was taking into the study. We now recognize that language as misleading, since it gave the impression that the data analysis was explicitly guided by a predetermined conceptual structure. More recently, we've used the term "theoretical scaffolding" to refer to this aspect so as to de-link it from data analysis while sustaining the emphasis on foregrounding the study with scholarly positioning.

There are two critical elements to scaffolding a study. The first element is the review of literature—the part where you come to know and draw conclusions about the "state of the science" in relation to the clinical problem you are concerned with. This allows you to confirm or challenge your initial hunch that the problem is worth studying in the first place, gives you insight as to who has already studied it, how they have gone about it, what problems they've encountered, and what sorts of conclusions they have reached so far. The second element of scaffolding has to do with working out what it is that you will be bringing into your own study. This will require that you account for the theoretical "baggage" you bring into the study—the disciplinary and theoretical ideas that have brought you to this point, the aspects of yourself and your thinking that will play a significant role in shaping what it is that this study becomes.

Conducting a Literature Review

Literature reviews have changed dramatically over the course of my own career, and the skill of sorting through an increasing array of accessible sources has become a science in itself (Booth, 2005; Sanders, 2005). While electronic indexing and retrieval systems have made it possible to access thousands of relevant sources very rapidly, they have created their own set of new challenges to those who aspire to becoming conversant with their field of study and to ensure that their own research efforts will be appropriately received within that body of knowledge.

Beyond what we might consider general good practice as regards reviewing literature for the purpose of adding useful scholarly contributions to it—a process that is well supported by most academic libraries and well-referenced within the literature—the elements of interpretive description that play a role in shaping a literature review have to do with its requirement for scaffolding, or locating oneself substantively, theoretically, and within a disciplinary orientation. Included here are some recommendations for things to consider in that context.

Finding Literature

Using an internet search engine these days, there are few topics on which the amateur computer user cannot find thousands of sources within a nanosecond. However, the business of finding the right sources, and being confident that one has a grasp on them, is quite a different matter. One of the frustrations of many academic leaders within this current context is that we may have a generation of students who are brilliant at using electronic technologies, but spend no time in actual libraries. While this observation may reflect a form of sentimental nostalgia for how things used to be, I think it also derives from a conviction that the library used to signify a place for tedious searches and spontaneous discoveries.

The Impact of the Internet The world of knowledge is currently accessed primarily through "keywords," and it is important to understand the limitations that this selection mechanism imposes. Keywords have been created within various disciplines to name the taxonomy of possible substantive subgroupings, and to become the primary search vehicle. For keywords to operate in the intended manner, some agreement as to which terms will become "key" is reached. Since keywords therefore reflect the "standard" state of conceptualization within a field at any given time, they can be a force of resistance against the kind of conceptual (and concept-labeling) change that is characteristic of a dynamic body of inquiry. Unfortunately, because authors tend to want others to easily locate their work, they may be inclined to revert to keyword choices that don't quite reflect what is new and different about their piece of the puzzle. Furthermore, most journals and referencing systems strictly limit the number of keywords that can be associated with any one piece of scholarship. Therefore, overreliance on keywords—especially when they produce large volumes of literature—has become a significant problem for many scholars.

The ease of access to internet and database sources also creates something of a barrier to the modern researcher. When thousands of sources can be accessed in seconds, it takes real courage to commit time and effort to seeking out what might or might not augment the study. What this means is that there is a preponderance of internet-accessible sources bolstering much of current research, and the kinds of knowledge that aren't quite so accessible tend to be ignored. In my view, this does create a skew in what people are inclined to think about a field, and can lead to problematic claims about the state of a science. I therefore encourage my own students to develop a wider repertoire of search resources to augment what they are likely to find electronically.

Expanding and Refining Your Search   First, you really do have to immerse yourself within the field while you are searching. While reading is an obvious starting point, there are many ways to augment that. If possible, try to participate in scholarly conferences in your field. Often a day or two listening to other scholars can be extraordinarily helpful in orienting you to the current problems within a field, to the way in which various groups of scholars are attempting to resolve them, and to the ideas that are new or controversial. As you read, you will also find that you are able to refine your capacity to recognize patterns within the literature, familiarize yourself with common understandings and spot variations, and make note of the authors who have been acknowledged as having made important contributions to that topic. Don't forget to read reference lists, and work at detecting who seems to be regularly cited as foundational to the field, who gets cited when certain biases or perspectives are being advanced, and the range of sources that scholars have been drawing from. This intellectual exercise may hurt at first, but consider it as a "warm-up" exercise for the pattern recognition process you'll be using when you get to data analysis.

Second, there are disciplinary groundings that may be requisite to your understanding of why certain kinds of scholarship are evolving in the way that they are. Because we all inevitably read outside of our own discipline, we encounter ideas that may be open to considerable misunderstanding if taken out of context. While none of us can be masters in all disciplines, I think it behooves the modern scholar to develop a reading familiarity with the basic elements and foundational concepts underlying the disciplines within which he or she is likely to read. The nurse drawing from research conducted by psychologists, for example, may not appreciate the subtle implications of language cues and foundational assumptions within a particular study, just as the psychologist may not be able to make sense of why the nurse research-er has assumed a practice utility to nongeneralizable findings. Fortu-nately, most disciplines have excellent "101" textbooks that are readily accessible in university libraries, and these can become an important beginning source of synthesis of the history and structure of the field. Often, a relatively quick review through the contents and introductory remarks will go a long way to "locating" a disciplinary orientation. As an alternative, various course outlines for such introductory courses can be found on the internet.

A third approach is to explore what has been called "grey literature" (Benzies, Premji, Hayden, & Serrett, 2006). When much of the literature is so readily accessible, it becomes quite easy to convince yourself that anything less accessible is unlikely to be important. Thus dissertations, policy reports, government "white papers," consensus conference reports, and other forms of important understanding can be prematurely dismissed. While an abbreviated search may be necessary in some instances of scholarship, if you are doing doctoral dissertation research on a topic, you will want to have an authoritative confidence that you really do know what is going on in your field, and have a solid grasp on its history and trajectory. For this reason, you will want to ensure that your search is as extensive as is humanly possible, and take the extra trouble to track down and reflect on potentially relevant nontraditional sources.

This brings us back to the library. Although the tedium of the manual search process had its drawbacks, it did create the climate in which the researcher was inclined to maximize efficiency by glancing through journal tables of contents over a period of several years, and to gaze at bookshelves within the same "region" as the books one was specifically seeking. These kinds of focused engagements often created the context in which new discoveries were made, tangentially related but fascinating knowledge was brought to light, and the mind was stimulated by the pervasive atmosphere of ideas. Many scholars have found that certain books just "leapt off the shelves" or that certain articles unrelated to what they thought they were searching for triggered a new and productive line of thinking. Thus, the library experience remains one that is precious to an earlier generation of researchers, and which many feel should not be lost.

Sorting and Organizing Literature

Once you have located sources (an operation that never ends in the dynamic and evolving research world, and operates in an entirely iterative manner with the organizational process), you have to decide what to do with them. In this, you will likely be guided by your research problem and the question that is forming in your mind in relation to it. Of course one's initial priority is typically trying to determine whether someone else has actually conducted the exact study one is anticipating doing, and so one organizational strategy is to sort the sources into the degree of proximity (conceptually, methodologically, or chronologically) to one's specific focus.

As you make a series of choices about literature to select or reject in this manner, you will likely find yourself swayed in various directions as regard what is and isn't relevant. It is quite important to keep notes on the decisions you make (not necessarily in reference to specific sources, but to groupings of them) so that you can retrace your logic later in the event that you need to expand your review beyond the more narrow scope you may have set. While some may find themselves prematurely rejecting sources that don't seem directly on target because of a desire to manage the volume of material, others will find that they are reluctant to put anything aside for fear that it may become useful at some point in the process. By reflecting on what sort of mental attitude you characteristically hold in this part of the process, you may well reveal an important insight about how you'll sort and organize data once in the field, and so it is useful to pay careful attention to these personal matters of process.

There is no question that setting boundaries on what you will actually use is necessary in this age of information explosion. And how you set those boundaries is a matter of considerable variation. While a prescriptive guide that will suit the needs of all studies is inconceivable, some general guidelines may help as you create and document your own decision trail.

First, some authors limit their searches to current knowledge, such as research conducted over an arbitrarily chosen time period such as the most recent five-year period (since this is easily accomplished by most database limits, it is easy to understand the appeal!). While this can be a useful first step to ascertain what's going on at the moment, I'd strongly suggest that you avoid this as a general search strategy. Most fields of study have an important history and a trajectory—who first used a certain conceptual term to reference a particular set of ideas or observations and what prompted that first usage, which disciplines or academic "camps" seem to have taken it up, what competing conceptualizations have emerged since it was first introduced, and so on.

While you might gain some impressions about these historical developments from the introductory and literature review sections of more recent authors, it will be important to judge for yourself from the primary and subsequent material. Unless you have access to a full understanding of what went into the making of a literature review of any published author, it is unwise to take his or her claims about the literature at face value. There are countless documented instances of misinterpretations of original sources that have been repeated over and over by subsequent authors, and you will want to ensure that future readers will not identify you with that form of sloppy scholarship. Indeed, ensuring that you have accessed and read the primary sources upon which your study relies is a hallmark of good science.

Another temptation can be to limit yourself to certain journals—most typically those within your discipline and with which you have some familiarity. While this might be appropriate if your topic is explicitly and exclusively disciplinary knowledge development, this kind of limit on a clinical topic about which others might well have written could significantly reduce your credibility in the field. One way to think this through is to look through a few sources within a related discipline to ascertain the way in which that discipline is dealing with the issue. You may be able to determine that, for example, in relation to your topic, there is a current lively debate going on within social anthropology, but the psychologists tend to have coalesced around a particular narrow perspective. In general, it becomes important not to discount what might have arisen from other disciplines until you've done a cursory sampling of it and developed a feel for the flavor of the product.

A third option that some people select is distinguishing research (data-based) from nonresearch literature. Again, doing so can be helpful in orienting you to who has been studying what, but you may miss out on some important synthesis papers or informed reviews that would help you considerably. Indeed, if systematic reviews, critical literature summaries, or other similar kinds of writing are available to you—either directly on your topic or on closely related topics—you will do well to read and consider them. A variation on this theme is to select studies that are qualitative rather than those that use combined or quantitative approaches. This strategy may have been sensible in an earlier era in which the two "paradigms" of research were considered antithetical, but it is quite counterproductive in the current context to lack familiarity with the entire field into which one is attempting to introduce new knowledge. While all researchers may have certain methods and traditions within which they are more comfortable reading, it is important to possess, at some level, a reading understanding of the full range of scholarship that is going on within the field that is to be the focus of your research. As you sort and organize you'll become well aware that, among scholarly journals, there can be a wide range of formats and quality criteria. You may wish to familiarize yourself with the most high-impact journals and those whose editorial review processes are most rigorous so that you can add another perspective to what might be considered strong or weak research within the field.

With current access techniques, the most readily accessible information about most scholarly papers is the abstract. Abstracts have become an excellent tool for the initial sorting process, in that they can provide you with sufficient information to know whether a paper is likely to be relevant to you, and if so, what "grouping" of relevant knowledge it will most likely contribute to. However, it is essential to understand that the abstract is not a substitute for the full paper—a point that all who have generated abstracts for their own studies will appreciate. While there may be occasions on which reference to an abstract alone would be sufficient (such as when you are providing a list of "kinds" of study, without commenting on their nature or quality in any way), all sources that have any potential utility in scaffolding your own study must be read in the original. Most academics have access to libraries within which this is easily accomplished electronically. In more challenging circumstances, if there really is no library access available to you, sometimes you can locate a paper by contacting the author directly for a "reprint."

Interpreting and Writing Up Your Literature Review

Typically, newer researchers need assistance with figuring out how to deal with the mountains of information that they have accessed. While one might long for a mechanistic and technical way to deal with it, there is absolutely no substitute for interpretation and reasoning in this stage of the process. It is therefore important to think about the kind of literature review that you are trying to produce and to transform that sorted and organized pile of sources into a logical sequence of ideas (Russell, 2005). A critical aspect of this step is to keep in mind your research question. While it may change or become refined before the end of your literature review process, it will be the instrument that keeps you on track and prevents you from shifting away from the core focus and onto the attractive side issues that you are certain to find within the literature.

Options in Writing a Literature Review Having immersed yourself in the literature, you will be well aware that there are multiple options for conceptualizing literature and writing it up. And so an early step must be to clarify in your own mind what kind of a literature review suits your purpose. While there may be practical considerations to keep in mind (such as the expected standards within your discipline, the programmatic requirements if you are conducting the research for a graduate degree), the kind of literature review that will best support an interpretive description is one that

- grounds the study within the existing knowledge,
- offers critical reflection on what exists and what does not, and
- offers commentary on the strengths and weaknesses within the overall body of knowledge.

In some disciplines, particularly those dominated by a more conventional scientific ethos, the expected form of a literature review is to write up, in a logical (usually chronological) sequence, a summary of key design elements of each of the related studies and then to attempt to expose their weaknesses. The conclusion of this kind of literature review tends to be that there have been flaws in the approaches of all prior researchers and this new study is designed to correct them. While that is a useful logic model for the kind of science for which it is intended, it is quite inappropriate for the requirements of an interpretive description.

Instead, the literature review that supports the need for an interpretive description will be one that explicitly documents what is (or seems to be) known and the nature of the inquiries upon which we have come to that knowledge. While it is quite likely that you have entered the field because you suspect there is more to be known, the best justification for additional study will derive from thoughtful and respectful consideration of what scholars have been doing in relation to the topic, what methods they have been employing in order to try to ascertain better understandings about aspects of the problem, and what kinds of understandings those methods may have led them to develop.

Orienting the Literature Review to Your Research Problem An important consideration in writing a literature review, no matter what kind of review you decide on, is the matter of conceptualizing or grouping bodies of literature and themes within it. In general, you are likely to find that some aspects of the literature are best dealt with as "bodies" of literature, and others may be best addressed as individual contributions. The kinds of literature that may well be summarized fairly generally will be by groups of authors who have been following a similar inquiry path, communities of scholars who have taken a particular stance on an issue, or even disciplinary groups that have formed coherent perspectives or orientations to the topic. As with all aspects of inductive reasoning, it may take you some time in the literature to get a "feel" for which are the ideas of common knowledge within the field that you could reference summarily, and which are the ideas that are sufficiently novel or controversial to warrant more detailed attention. Depending on the nature and substance of the available literature, you have a number of options for organizing your material, such as chronologically, by discipline, by theoretical perspective, by method, or by "closeness" to the actual clinical issue at hand.

Before deciding on your overall organizing structure, you'll want to consider what kind of an argument each of the available sequencing options could build. For example, a chronological sequence would be appropriate if there has been a direct line of development from the initial research to the present day, and your study is explicitly designed to build upon it. However, if your study is designed to flesh out our understanding from the perspective of those with experiential knowledge as to why there are major discrepancies between disciplines or perspectives on a topic, then you are most likely to illustrate that most effectively with a disciplinary or perspectival sequence.

Concluding the Literature Review   The strategic objective for which a literature review is enacted is setting the stage for a good argument that further research is needed and that research using the general approach you intend would make a valuable contribution. If you have effectively organized and sequenced your literature review to build logically to this conclusion, you are well on your way to the next step of actually articulating the design specifics.

If the field seems to be one in which knowledge is well-established and accepted, then you will have to be able to identify at least one problem associated with accepting that understanding in order to justify the need for your new study. Often, researchers entering the field will find that they have misinterpreted what exists until they've conducted the thorough literature search, and it can be discouraging to discover your topic is not as important as you thought it might be. However, having read and reviewed the relevant literature, you'll also have paid careful attention to the conclusions that your predecessors have made as to the future directions for research that would advance the field. From these informed conclusions, you can very often find inspiration for refining your angle of attention on the problem so that it regains relevance.

If the field is one in which there has been relatively little study, you'll have to think about how you are going to justify devoting time

TEXT BOX 3.1

Caregiving in the Cultural Context

Using an interpretive description approach, Cioffi sought a better understanding of what it is like for family members to stay with their relatives in acute care hospital wards when they are of a nondominant cultural background. Cioffi had noticed that, despite the commitment of nurses to involving family as the core of care, there was very little recognition in the literature of the particular challenge associated with the culturally diverse population in this regard. From interviews with family members, Cioffi learned that their experience involved engaging in a number of in-hospital roles, often involving interpretation and advocacy. They were extremely aware of ward rules that arose from hospital policy and tried to take them into consideration. They also experienced a variety of personal concerns, ranging from discomfort with situations they witnessed to being unable to manage some aspects of their relative's care and being worried about the future. These findings served as a basis from which Cioffi was able to question some of the typical ways that nurses negotiate family access to the patient and communicate expectations of the helping role that families play in the caregiving context.

Cioffi, J. (2006). Culturally diverse family members and their hospitalized relatives in acute care wards: A qualitative study. *Australian Journal of Advanced Nursing, 24*(1), 15–20.

and effort to the topic. It may be one that has arisen within the clinical practice context but not yet reached the attention of researchers within the field, or it may be one that is sufficiently obscure or context-specific that it has not found its way into importance. The absence of prior study does not in and of itself justify the need for new research. Rather, your challenge will be to conclude your literature review with a solid case for this new line of inquiry, building upon what is known and not known in relation to similar topics, and also upon what can be concluded about the importance of the issue within clinical practice.

In order for a literature review to substantiate the need for an interpretive description, it will have to conclude that there is something related to patterns within human activity (experience, behavior, or consciousness) that would flesh out what is currently known and allow us to better understand the phenomenon within the practice context. In other words, you must credibly conclude that there is relevant knowledge to which actors within the field have experiential access that has not yet been sufficiently documented, described, or interpreted to make that level of knowledge useful in some manner to a discipline's activity or project. Essentially, you need to establish what we wish to know, where that knowledge may reside, and why it matters.

Clarifying the Theoretical Forestructure

The second element of scaffolding a study has to do with "locating" yourself as a researcher within the field and the theoretical world that surrounds it. In contrast to the motivation inherent in most quantitative designs which seek to neutralize any influence that the researcher might bring to the research process, interpretive description, like all qualitative approaches, explicitly recognizes and capitalizes on the researcher as instrument. This does not mean that you get to do whatever you feel, but rather that your actions and thinking do play a meaningful role in shaping the nature and outcome of your inquiry, and in determining the manner in which your eventual research findings will or will not make a contribution that others in your field deem credible, and so you need to thoughtfully account for them.

There are several linked elements to this theoretical forestructure:

- locating your theoretical allegiances on entering the study,
- locating yourself within a discipline, and
- locating your personal relationship to the ideas you hold.

Each element represents an intellectual exercise you need to engage in as part of writing up your research proposal (and deciding what to put into it) and before you enter the field to collect data. While there are few absolute rules around forestructuring, the key is an integrity of purpose not only within yourself, but between yourself and your project, and with your eventual audience. Because, as a researcher, your mind and your personhood are integrally involved in what you will accomplish, it is only with some honest reflection on these elements that you can ensure that the research products you generate are true to your purpose and become meaningful empirical contributions.

Locating Theoretical Allegiances

Because interpretive description locates itself outside of the social science theoretical tradition, it does not require that all studies be explicitly located within one or another formal theorization. As with "normal science," in which the legitimacy of a research question is entirely dependent on its relationship to those that have gone before, the social science tradition has evolved in such a manner that the theoretical links between scholarly projects must be made explicit (Sandelowski, 1993b, 2000). Therefore, in a social science proposal or report, we typically see language that "cues" the informed disciplinary reader into understanding that the tradition of certain scholars is being followed and that specific strands of thinking are being taken up. This theoretical positioning ensures that the findings will contribute to a larger theoretical project of concern to the discipline.

For example, when an author references "symbolic interactionism" as a theoretical positioning, one recognizes that he or she is working in the tradition of Mead (1934) and Blumer (1969), emphasizing interpretation as an essential human response, rejecting behaviorism and other branches of psychology, and explicitly concerned with the signs and symbols with which people signify meaning within their interactions with one another ("semiotics"). Further, one might rightly assume the intention to use grounded theory methodology to uncover what is assumed to constitute a "basic social process" as yet not uncovered or articulated so that we can more fully understand that aspect of human meaning-making through interaction. If the research report did not take up these issues in a serious manner, the reader might consider the author to have inappropriately "tossed in" the reference without understanding its meaning to the target audience. In contrast, while authors such as Blumer and Mead contributed quite broadly to knowledge and one might justifiably wish to reference them in relation to different ideas, their association with this strand of thinking has become so entrenched that it would require firm and explicit negation of that association to communicate to the reader that the common linkage is not intended. Thus, one does not enter into the business of citing authorities lightly, since it is within these citations that the astute reader will discern theoretical affinities, contradictions in perspective, and signals as to the tradition to which the new inquiry is intending to contribute.

Often, as with the above example, the theoretical cues reflect methodological as well as substantive information. For instance, when language such as "lifeworld" or "lived experience" is used to frame a study, readers will normally anticipate a phenomenological orientation and a methodological option that is consistent with that tradition. While ethnographers certainly gather data on lifeworlds and lived experiences, they generally refer to these concepts using alternative linguistic signifiers. Often scholars within a particular scholarly community will immediately recognize certain terminology as "loaded" with meaning while others in different academic groupings may not. Your job is to understand the academic culture into which you are attempting to make inroads, to learn to speak its language fluently and intelligently, and to begin to understand how the assumptions and beliefs underlying its linguistic cues are similar or different from those of other knowledge communities. Although it can be quite tempting to "throw in" obscure or intriguing references you may have encountered in your reading, it is important to recognize that, unless you really do intend to take them seriously and have them explicitly guide design and application decisions in your research, their inclusion in a superficial manner may harm your standing with important audiences. A casual reference to Michel Foucault, for example, might communicate to informed scholars a very explicit set of understandings about the dynamics of knowledge and power that one would expect to see showcased prominently within the findings. If you don't intend that, or aren't sure, you might do well to avoid complicating your life. Thus, ensuring that you are as aware as you can be of the language cues within your field and their implications for communicating your relationship to various theoretical perspectives becomes an important part of crafting a credible research proposal and project.

Locating the Discipline

Each discipline can be said to have what it considers its profound and burning question—the ultimate reason that justifies the existence of a scholarly community. According to Michael Quinn Patton, sociology's burning question is something like, What holds society together? For psychology it is, Why do individuals think, feel, and act as they do? For economics, the question becomes, How are resources produced and distributed? Biologists ask, What is the nature and variety of life? And agriculturists wonder, How do we produce food? (Patton, 2002, p. 216) Although Patton acknowledges that reducing multifaceted disciplines to a single question oversimplifies their inherent complexity, his point is that understanding the fundamental question that binds one's discipline together permits clarity and focus in distinguishing one's disciplinary angle of vision from that of any other.

Although the issue has long attracted controversy, and there are diverse philosophical standpoints within the tradition itself (Schwandt, 1997), phenomenological frameworks typically required that the researcher strive toward *epoché,* making every effort to set aside preconceived ideas prior to entry into the experiential lifeworld of another. This "bracketing" or suspension of the "natural attitude" created the conditions for discerning the core "essence" of the phenomenon under study (Husserl, 1929/1975; Miller & Crabtree, 1999a). This idea has tremendous appeal to the study of deeply felt subjective experience in such contexts as loneliness or grief, for example, and we might fully appreciate the value of embarking on study of the phenomenon through the filter of the research participant's subjectivity rather than prematurely developed personal experiential "insights." However, a naïve attraction to this idea has also led a number of qualitative health researchers to presume that it is legitimate to study a health-related question without proper appreciation of the current state of knowledge affecting the field. This problem of the "blank slate" is one that seems entirely inconsistent with the advancement of disciplinary knowledge, and its misapplication has contributed to what others have noted as a misuse of phenomenological approaches in answering questions pertaining to human experience and meaning (Anderson, 1989; Morse, 1994c; Ray, 1994; Schultz & Meleis, 1988; Thorne, 1991).

As a form of disciplinary knowledge development, interpretive description would require sufficient grounding in the discipline to be able to discern its scope and boundaries, its angle of vision on problems of concern, and its philosophical underpinnings in relation to what constitutes knowledge. This stance requires not only that one "owns up" to one's disciplinary heritage, but also explicitly positions a new research question within it. Thus, an important element in the forestructuring of any study is to consider its disciplinary nature, to consider the manner in which it aligns itself with the knowledge and practice of the discipline, and to sort out how that will be made apparent within the research design and eventual write-up.

Having reviewed many qualitative studies for such purposes as metasynthesis, I have been intrigued with the various ways in which disciplinary orientation creeps into qualitative studies, even when the author had not intended to make it transparent (Thorne, Joachim, Paterson, & Canam, 2002). It can be detected within the bodies of literature that are included in the review, the language that is employed within the report, the characteristic styles with which the design issues are elaborated or obscured. What concerns me is that, in their effort to "locate" the specific theorists they have been reading or the theoretical affinities they have formed, researchers often forget to consider the implications of their disciplinary orientation upon their work, and in so doing, neglect an important element in its overall impact and quality.

From my perspective, recognizing that one's very enthusiasm for a topic derives directly from a disciplinary interest in it becomes an essential aspect of the research forestructure and grounding. Awareness that this is the case will afford the researcher a level of insight later on when it comes to drawing conclusions on the basis of the study and in articulating any implications or recommendations that derive from the findings. Thus, I am suggesting that we consider discipline "as theory" in the sense of understanding the manner in which it will inevitably shape

- what it is we decide to observe in the field,

- what we see when we make those observations, and

- what sense we begin to make of the observations as they progress.

Having commented on the role of theory and discipline, it becomes important to distinguish disciplinary perspective from theory development within the discipline. In some instances, research questions directly derive from disciplinary theorizing. So, for example, a psychologist might wonder whether a cognitive or a behavioral approach would better serve the process of changing health behavior habits within certain populations. In order to gain clarity about the nature and scope of the intended study, it will be important to sort out whether the study is about better understanding the clinical population through comparing two distinct intervention approaches, or whether the study is about better understanding the theoretical perspective underlying the intervention by testing it out on additional populations. This complex interrelationship between clinical and theoretical motivation is a particular problem where integrity of method and design logic are concerned.

As a method for generating knowledge pertaining to clinically derived phenomena, interpretive description explicitly locates itself within the applied disciplinary domain. It departs from the conventional methods designed for disciplines whose object is theorizing, and addresses a distinct need for inquiry approaches where certain kinds of clinical problems or populations warrant inquiry that describes and interprets patterns of experience, action, or expression. As such, it is "atheoretical" but with explicit recognition that the nature of the problem derives directly from a set of ideas and structures about practice disciplines that may have theoretical elements but are not themselves theory. "Theory building" disguised as clinical research will not be well served by this inquiry approach, since it becomes an inherently circular argument. If you enter an interpretive descriptive study with the intention of confirming a particular perspective, your mind will inevitably be drawn toward observations and interpretations that support it and away from those that render it more problematic. Thus this distinction between theory-driven research and research that is structured in such a manner as to account for and acknowledge a disciplinary orientation is an important one that must be carefully and thoughtfully handled.

Positioning the Researcher Within the Ideas

A hallmark of qualitative research is that it explicitly capitalizes on the person who is considered the "instrument" of the research. Consequently, the quality of the process and the product are inexorably dependent on the integrity of that researcher in accounting for the mechanisms by which the eventual outcomes can be judged (Lipson, 1989; Purkis, 1994). While academic and personal integrity are clearly fundamental to the spirit of qualitative scholarship (Knafl, 1994), the integrity we are concerned with here is more an intellectual integrity in the sense of having "located" oneself—or the specific relevant elements that make up that complex self—within this particular research project.

Since interpretive description is designed as a method for those who wish to study problems whose origins are the needs of the clinical field, the disciplinary orientation helps us understand what the motivation for the study entails and what the potential audience for any new knowledge that arises from the study might be. While the impact of the study may not be limited to that audience, its particular needs are unlikely to drift far from the consciousness of the researcher, and therefore deserve a formal place in the "positioning."

Depending on the specific topic, it may be of considerable importance to further locate the specific kinds of concerns that contributed to the generation of the area of interest. Were patterns observed among hospital patients with a particular condition? Did clinic staff begin to report a particular kind of family response to a situation? Were there particular kinds of clients who seemed less well served by standard protocols than others? These matters of the genesis of the inspiration for the research are important to acknowledge in setting up a study, since they will reveal something of the motivation and bias of the researcher and become a fixed point against which it becomes possible to determine whether data collection and analysis are either informed or skewed by these earliest conceptions.

TEXT BOX 3.2

Adapting to Kidney Failure

An experienced nephrology nurse who had struggled to find relevant information to assist with meeting the distinctive care needs of patients whose kidney failure related to pre-existing diabetes, Ravenscroft used interpretive description to better understand the dynamics of their experience. This author found that the advent of kidney failure was distressing for these individuals, significantly augmenting the extent to which illness intruded into their daily lives, particularly in the context of time and intimate relationships. The findings further documented the challenge patients encountered with adjusting to this new chronic condition, including their efforts to maintain control over some elements of their personal lives and their attempts to sustain hope. On the basis of these findings, Ravenscroft proposes that ensuring continuity of care and the promotion of collaborative patient-health care provider relationships within the hemodialysis clinic setting may assist these individuals in their attempts to normalize living and support their attempts to maintain as positive an outlook as possible.

Ravenscroft, E. F. (2005). Diabetes and kidney failure: How individuals with diabetes experience kidney failure. *Nephrology Nursing Journal, 32*(4), 502–509.

The researcher may also have been powerfully influenced by certain ideas, theories, or inquiry approaches prior to or during the process of bringing the initial curiosity to the point of becoming a formal research question. Graduate students may well have been inspired by particularly charismatic teachers, clinical researchers by compelling new theoretical stances, or established scholars by the specific theoretical claims that served us well in prior studies. As human beings with inquiring minds, we are often quite susceptible to the most recent good book we read or lecture we attended. Thus, in the case of each of these issues, it is important to surface, acknowledge, and reflect upon what ideas we hold that may be influencing us in the design and implementation of this project.

We have already discussed why interpretive description explicitly distinguishes itself from qualitative research whose primary object is theorizing, and is most comfortable within a somewhat atheoretical context. However, no human being is immune from theoretical influence (and bias), and therefore the way in which this susceptibility is handled involves explicit recognition and understanding, so that it influences the research in ways that are consistent with integrity to an inductive reasoning process that generates findings that are well grounded within data.

In her discussion of the application of classic qualitative technique to qualitative description, Sandelowski helpfully distinguishes between full-on adoption of specific ideas and a less "pure" situation in which those ideas shape what she calls the "hues, tones and texture" of what we study (2000, p. 337). By differentiating between claims that are made with respect to whole perspectives and those that are made in relation to the specific elements that are being applied, she shows how drawing upon a range of methods and perspectives, even when apparently contradictory, can be quite consistent with solid qualitative inquiry. When we understand how to effectively convey our relationship with the ideas we are referencing, we convey an integrity of purpose that will not be confused with misuse of methods or erroneous claims.

The important distinction between ways of communicating our particular relationship to ideas can be illustrated with the application of any one of the "standpoints" that increasingly appear within our qualitative research literature. For example, feminism is an idea that is commonly referenced in relation to aspects of health that involve gender (and also often those that do not). For the researcher entering a study on a women's health topic, there is a significant difference between declaring oneself to "be" a feminist and acknowledging that some aspect of feminist thought will have influenced one's work. Whether one is or is not a feminist in private life is not particularly relevant to the research project, unless, of course, it is likely to be significant to the process of gaining entry into the field, in which case its influence becomes a significant limitation within the data analysis process. If one claims a piece of research "is" a feminist study, then one has made a commitment to a whole series of design and methodological claims (Thorne & Varcoe, 1988) that privilege a certain predetermined world view over the perspectives that may arise within the field during the data collection process. However, if one claims that some aspect of the study has been "informed" by feminist thought (perhaps the importance of the question, the scope of the literature that has been reviewed, some specific design considerations), then the relationship to the theoretical idea has been presented in such a manner as to lend integrity to the research process and create the conditions under which a high-quality interpretive description becomes achievable.

In general, if ideas, thoughts, perspectives, or personal experiences are going to influence the angle of vision that you are taking into a study, it is always best to confess them and ensure that you appropriately manage and account for them. However, in this context, I must admit that I am not a fan of the overblown extensive personal reflection that does sometimes appear in the write-ups of certain qualitative reports. One hopes that the researcher is primarily fascinated with the subject rather than the self, and the quality of the findings will be inherently suspect if there is too much of the author within the product. While there may be a place for autoethnography in the world, readers of interpretive description (as with most qualitative studies) will be taking up your study because they share an enthusiasm for solving the clinical problem, not because they want private information about your life and your experience conducting the project. So the appropriate "positioning" that you do in relation to your study will be that which is explicitly necessary to understand your motivations, your biases, and your consequent angle of interpretive inquiry.

By bringing together the conclusions about the field that you have drawn from your literature review, and presenting that in the context of the theoretical, disciplinary, and personal forestructure that will be shaping both the design decisions and analytic maneuvers you will be making, you will have effectively scaffolded your qualitative inquiry. Your reader (that mythical "judge" we all have looking over our shoulders as we work) will be appropriately informed as to what you—the research instrument—bring into the study and the manner in which that instrument will influence what will happen and what may be discovered. From this base, you will be well positioned to build a credible and defensible interpretive description project whose conclusions follow logically from the original objectives that you set for yourself, and whose results have the potential to be meaningful. You want to enter your study comfortable with who you are and what you've revealed about yourself, and well armed with the humility that it takes to realize that the extent to which you succeed in minimizing the unintended impact you have on the process of your research will in large measure determine your ability to produce a high-quality research product.

Framing a Study Design

As is evident from the discussion in previous chapters, interpretive description does not prescribe an exact way to go about a study, but rather represents itself as a design logic model whereby the kinds of qualitative studies that are typically generated on behalf of the applied disciplines can be designed and enacted with meaningful results. In this way, it serves as a framework within which various data collection and analytic strategies can be usefully employed, as long as their use remains consistent with the overall logic and intent of the study. The excellent work of so many social and applied scientists to generate research techniques, strategies, and mechanisms becomes a wonderful resource for interpretive description. What is required, therefore, is an understanding of the implications of the techniques—where they came from and what they are used for within their original context.

Like most qualitative research methods, interpretive description arose out of an expressed need for an alternative way to generate certain species of knowledge. It reflected not so much a vision for the future as a strategy for legitimizing the very fine research that was being produced within the discipline of nursing for which there really was no other name (Morse, 1989a). Like all of my colleagues at that time, I too had been constructing my research findings within design language that did not in its entirety fit my needs. In various incarnations of my program of research, I had used phenomenology, grounded theory, ethnography, and naturalistic inquiry as the structural frame within which I explained how I conducted my study and articulated the way in which my findings emerged. However, none of these had proven a perfect fit and—if truth be told—I could see significant methodological flaws within my enactment of these methods precisely because I was grounding my studies in clinical issues rather than advancing theorizing. By "naming" interpretive description as a disciplinary approach to qualitative research, my coauthors and I created a point of legitimation for others who had similarly been wrestling with available method. What we did not do was generate new or original design options; rather, we simply created a rationale for linking them together in a coherent and defensible manner that would more suitably meet the knowledge-generation needs of our applied health discipline.

Foundational Underpinnings of Interpretive Description

In this chapter and the next, we'll focus on issues of research design—the kinds of issues one needs to make decisions about in order to complete a research proposal and justify entering the field for data collection and analysis. What this chapter will reveal is not an explicit prescription, but rather an invitation to the reader to engage in an exploration of what some of the options might be for qualitative inquiry about disciplinary problems—inquiry that will have several common features because they are bound by the same set of assumptions about human experience and about the nature and production of knowledge pertaining to it. Interpretive description studies

- are conducted in as naturalistic a context as possible in a manner that is respectful of the comfort and ethical rights of all participants,
- explicitly attend to the value of subjective and experiential knowledge as one of the fundamental sources of clinical insight,
- capitalize on human commonalities as well as individual expressions of variance within a shared focus of interest,
- reflect issues that are not bounded by time and context, but attend carefully to the time and context within which the current expressions are enacted,
- acknowledge a socially "constructed" element to human experience that cannot be meaningfully separated from its essential nature,
- recognize that, in the world of human experience, "reality" involves multiple constructed realities that may well be contradictory, and
- acknowledge an inseparable relationship between the knower and the known, such that the inquirer and the "object" of that inquiry interact to influence one another.

Because they understand the world in this particular way, practitioners of interpretive description enter their studies assuming that *a priori* theory cannot encompass these multiple realities; rather, they recognize that theory about a clinical phenomenon must emerge from or be grounded in that phenomenon.

These ideas, many of which are informed by key axioms within naturalistic inquiry tradition of Lincoln & Guba (1985), represent the epistemological foundation of interpretive description. Although interpretive description studies may differ one from another in relation to certain techniques for data collection and approaches to data analysis, these philosophical underpinnings ensure a coherence that distinguishes the products of interpretive description from those derived from blended approaches or from generic qualitative description.

Elements of Design

Interpretive description studies provide a thematic or integrative description of a phenomenon of clinical interest, and do so in a manner in which the disciplinary objects of the study are made explicit within the interpretations. To achieve this, interpretive description designs will, in various ways, search out and explore features or elements of a common issue, but will seek to render an understanding of them that honors their inherent complexity. In so doing, they will be structured so as to ensure that the inherent value of all expressed perceptions is recognized, without falling into the trap of assuming that what is perceived is always and necessarily "true." They will ground the interpretive, analytic conclusions that arise within the individual and collective representations of data, demonstrating the manner in which individual instances have contributed to a general pattern within the process.

While there will be a number of common elements to interpretive description designs, we would also anticipate a wide range of "flavors." For example, one researcher using interpretive description to study women involved with breast cancer advocacy groups might position the rationale for that study as being "informed" by the emphasis of hermeneutics on the intersection between public and private process. Another studying marginalized immigrant families within a particular community context might explicitly draw upon ethnographic techniques to guide the steps and substance of data collection. A third studying live birth following stillbirth might take advantage of some of the analytic procedures for thematic analysis within grounded theory methodology in order to explore for the presence of common social process issues among individual accounts. Thus, interpretive description exists as a coherent methodological framework within which a fairly wide range of options for design decisions can be enacted and justified.

Mapping Out the Plan

As all researchers know, there are two distinct processes in working out design—what you claim you will do and what actually happens. Ideally, these two processes are similar in most important regards; however, in the enactment of any study, and perhaps specifically a qualitative study, there are many decision points along the way that will shape the way in which the "best-laid plans" actually materialized in the real setting. In this chapter and the next, we'll discuss planning, and the decisions you will make with regard to such matters as data sources, sampling considerations, data collection methods, and credibility requirements. In subsequent chapters, a more in-depth discussion of the enactment of the complex processes of data collection and analysis will serve as a guide to considering some of the common pitfalls and challenges that even the most meticulous planner will often find once out in the "field."

Writing a Study Proposal

All scientific research begins with an explicit proposal. In the qualitative health context, this is typically a thesis/dissertation proposal (if you are a student) or a grant proposal (if you are an established researcher). What the proposal does is force you to name a problem of some relevance, think through the scaffolding of your study, make a strong case that it is worth doing, and outline a clear and explicit roadmap for how you will do it.

One of the best ways to conceptualize a proposal is to have the opportunity to read the proposals of others. While the enormity of a qualitative project can make your first experience quite daunting, there is a logic to it, and seeing how others have laid theirs out can provide you with some ideas and overall direction. There are also a number of excellent resources available in the literature to specifically guide you in the process of creating proposals for different purposes and audiences (Carey & Swanson, 2003; Connelly & Yoder, 2000; Knafl & Deatrick, 2005; J. A. Maxwell, 1998; Morse, 1994a; Patton, 2002; Sandelowski & Barroso, 2003c; Sandelowski, Davis, & Harris, 1989). What this brief chapter will do is orient you to the nature of the decisions you'll have to make about your study, and invite you to consider some of the approaches and strategies that have been found useful by others doing research within this framework.

Obtaining Ethical Approval

Another requirement of all qualitative research at this preliminary stage is ethical approval. While interpretive description studies rarely involve the potential for bodily harm or high-risk activity, it is a fundamental premise of modern research that the information that research "subjects" provide must be used in such a manner that their interests and needs are respected. Further, there is a profound understanding that information about people, and about groups, when interpreted or disseminated inappropriately, can significantly compromise people's interests (Giordano, O'Reilly, Taylor, & Dogra, 2007; Morse, 2005; Sieber, 1998). As we have learned from many classic situations, the potential harm to which research exposes people cannot be fully ameliorated by the singular element of obtaining informed consent.

While many of the "standard" requirements of informed consent and ethical research procedure can seem awkward within the qualitative context, scholars have found various ways to balance the "fluidity" of open-ended inquiry processes with the "rigidity" required by various ethical review boards (Lipson, 1994; Munhall, 1989). Newer researchers who do not have access to seasoned mentors in this regard will do well to consult the literature as well as make inquiries to their local ethics boards. Although the general principles of ethical procedure are common across jurisdictions, there are typically highly particular and specific requirements in each university or health authority context you may encounter.

Selecting Among Design Options

The basic design options of a study reveal a lot about your

- philosophical underpinnings,
- assumptions about the relationship between ideas and experience,
- perceptions of what kind of knowledge you are seeking,
- sense of the ultimate purpose in so doing.

Newer qualitative researchers sometimes enter a study with a vague sense that what they want to do is talk to certain people about a certain topic, but there is much more to consider when actually mapping out a design. Here we'll introduce some of the key considerations in what kind of data sources you might rely upon, how you might decide which representatives of those sources to engage with, what you might do with them when you find them, and what sense you will be able to make of it all. It can be confusing to think it all through, but having a clearly defensible plan, even if you have to make detours from it along the way, is fundamental to producing worthwhile results.

Deciding on Data Sources

Interviewing

Because finding ways to bring subjectively derived knowledge into the disciplinary armament is what draws most health care professionals into qualitative inquiry in the first place, it is no wonder that interviewing has become the primary source of data in so many fields of clinical qualitative inquiry. Indeed the predominance of subjective data, obtained through individual interviews has attracted considerable critique, and the hazards of overreliance on this particular form of understanding have been strongly debated within the literature (Nunkoosing, 2005; Sandelowski, 2002; Silverman, 1985). In the clinical health fields, interviewing is as familiar as breathing, and the kinds of subjectively inquisitive minds who turn to qualitative health problems often feel very comfortable in engaging "informants," thinking that their experience in clinical interviewing will have prepared them for the skill set required of the research interview. However, this can be an importantly erroneous assumption, and we'll discuss this later when reflecting on what happens in the process of data collection.

Interpretive description explicitly locates itself within a philosophical tradition that tells us—at least in matters involving human experience—the "more probable truths" (Johnson, 1996; Kikuchi & Simmons, 1996; Sandelowski, 1996) are those that we have arrived at using multiple angles of vision. In understanding a human clinical problem, we quickly recognize why teasing out a single measurable variable in order to quantify a complex phenomenon cannot effectively represent whole experience in context. However, in our enthusiasm to balance narrow perspectives with qualitative inquiries, we sometimes forget that subjectivity also has clear limits. If we consider our relationship to the "grand stories" of our own lives, those narratives we build about how key events occurred, we all recognize that subjective knowledge is shaped and constructed according to many masters—including ego, ideology, and social meaning. Although we are both fully competent and aware participants within a difficult family decision-making process, it is inevitable that my brother will recall the same event quite differently. We know that about how we live in the world, and yet we sometimes forget it in the world of qualitative health research, where the recollections of individuals about their traumatic or profound experiences can become reified into a form of a truth that seems incontestable (Nunkoosing, 2005; Sandelowski, 1991).

To some extent, this overreliance on subjective material as our closest approximation of "truth" derives from the extent to which we have relied upon phenomenology, which essentially studies entities for which there is no other material or social truth than the subjective. If I want to understand what it feels like to hear shocking news, or to try to climb out of depression, the only way in which I can come to "know" the essence of that experience is through the various mechanisms by which subjective experience, at its most basic, is rendered into a form that is accessible to my consciousness and reason. Poets, artists, storytellers, and phenomenologists all contribute to my capacity to have that experience vicariously and therefore to come to "know" it in a sense that is meaningful.

In contrast, despite its sincere commitment to tapping that form of knowledge, a great deal of qualitative inquiry is more about "empathizing" or "understanding" than it is about knowing in the existential sense, and this has created much of the departure from phenomenological tradition that we see today. We seek patterns and themes within subjective human experience not so much as to grasp its essence as to understand what we are likely to encounter in future clinical practice and to have some meaningful sensitivity around it. Thus, the deepest individual expression that can be captured on film or in print will certainly become part of what informs us in our practice, but it may also paralyze us into inaction or mislead us as to which aspects of that experience are unique to individuals rather than commonly shared. Thus, although interpretive description owes a great deal to phenomenological methods, it reflects a quite different attitude toward knowledge and knowing.

That said, there is still good reason for capitalizing on individual interviews as a useful core for the development of knowledge in relation to many of the clinical issues we encounter. If we want to understand what kinds of responses scleroderma patients encounter when they attempt to seek primary care with nonspecialist clinicians, our best bet is likely to ask a few of those patients and to systematically organize and make sense of any common elements. We know that interviewing one or two, we might get a feel for the issue quite quickly, but as clinicians we also know that we might well have tapped into those one or two who represent the more complacent or frustrated end of the spectrum. Thus, although the clinical case report has its honored place in medical literature, qualitative researchers tend to rely much more heavily on accounts that involve multiple people. We'll say more later about how to decide how many is sufficient.

Participant Observation

Next to interviewing, participant observation is the most common source of data for most qualitative health researchers. Again, its appeal is perhaps that it feels quite familiar. As practice-based professionals, we are comfortable being on the inside, and assume that "hanging out" in a purposeful manner can surface patterns and themes within what we observe.

Participant observation was designed as a way to get at people's thinking through understanding patterns in how they behaved. It is the primary tool of the ethnographer who is trying to make sense of the tacit understandings underlying the actions and behaviors of people from cultures with rule sets different from one's own. By watching in a careful and meticulous way, and systematically documenting what it is that we see, we can begin to appreciate the social structures under-lying what seems on the surface to be a curious action. A significant advantage of participant observation is that it allows the researcher to operate from a standpoint that is not overly influenced by subjectivi-ty—why people think they are doing things in the way that they are. While traditional ethnography typically combined participant observa-tion with key informant interviews, the intellectual "distance" that the anthropologist was encouraged to take from the ways of the culture was what permitted the possibility of useful theorizing. Indeed, being too close to the logic of the social groups that were being observed put the researcher at risk for suspicion of "going native" and the research products being discounted.

In the applied health research context, participant observation rais-es a number of important problems that must be taken into consider-ation. First, the clinical researcher has the problem of already having been socialized into "seeing" the field with a particular professional lens. The power of that lens, and its capacity to radically alter what you see and what sense you make of it, has been vividly captured, for ex-ample, in various accounts of seasoned clinicians who become patients (Sacks, 1984). This is not to say that clinicians are inherently insensi-tive to what the world looks like from the perspective of those who receive their care, but that the experience from the "other side" can be profoundly myth-shattering when it moves beyond the virtual and into the real. What this tells us is that it is not at all unproblematic to do par-ticipant observation in a world in which you already have familiarity and undoubtedly well-formed opinions, even if they lurk somewhere below the surface of what you can comfortably bring to consciousness. Thus, the task of the participant observer is to rigorously and systematically ensure that the lens through which you are looking is open, transparent, and clear, and the quality of your research product will depend entirely on how convincingly you can accomplish that. What that will mean is not simply claiming suspension of prior belief, but continuously challenging yourself to consider what else you might be missing, what alternative interpretations might pertain to what you are seeing. And, because the human mind does have a tendency to pattern and interpret on its own, and to convince itself of its conclusions, you will have to accept the possibility that what you conclude may expose you to a significant critique if your conclusions do not match the perspectives of others.

Focus Groups

The idea of bringing groups of people together and triggering a group engagement within a topic that then becomes a source of data derives from two distinct traditions, and it is important to understand something of that. One species of focus group arose from academic activity to promote revolutionary social change in South America (Fals-Borda & Rahman, 1991; Friere, 1970), and became a mechanism whereby the academic community could work in tandem with local groups to create a social movement and produce massive economic reform. This kind of focus group was designed specifically to galvanize communities into action because of the power that their shared knowledge could offer them once they had brought it to consciousness and recognized its potential. The other kind of focus group derived from North American market research, in which it was to the benefit of corporations to create a mechanism by which to understand public opinion. The idea here was that, rather than sampling individual opinions, which notoriously change under social pressure, to gather a group of individuals, expose them to a particular idea, and see what kind of consensus evolved within the social dynamic. In this way, focus groups were very much about using research to uncover or create shared perspective, rather than to pay serious attention to individual differences. This profound recognition of the effect of the group—considered a microcosm of society—is a hallmark of focus group methodology.

While bringing people with similar experiences together to exchange ideas is unquestionably a powerful tool for public opinion or social consciousness building, it is important to remember that not all health problems worthy of study inherently derive from an assumption of the dominance of social forces. Certainly when the health research has to do with mobilizing powerless consumer groups, or energizing leaders of disadvantaged demographic subsets in an "action research" approach, the focus group might well be the data collection strategy of choice. However, if the point of the research is to understand commonalities and diversities among people who have, for example, sought treatment for a particular disease condition, then the focus group might well be fundamentally wrong for your purpose.

Sadly, it would seem that qualitative health researchers sometimes look toward focus group designs as an apparently efficient way to gain interview data on larger numbers of individuals. However, since the group dynamic is the foundation of the focus group, inappropriate use of this technique can systematically obscure important perspectives and lead to dangerously wrong results. Among patients who have had a particular illness, for example, those who are the most ill or angry will inevitably be given the most airtime within a group discussion, as those who feel more privileged or lucky are easily silenced. Because focus groups are not the best context for individuals to freely "tell their own story" in any meaningful manner, they deprive the researcher of the more in-depth experiential variation that makes individual interviews so compelling. And because such groups capitalize on the social dynamic, they tend to wash out elements of the common experience that are not easily articulated or justified. By understanding what focus groups do and why you might use them, you can make thoughtful choices as to whether they will or will not serve the unique needs of your particular study.

Documentary and Other Collateral Data Sources

An often neglected data source is text that might expose you to subjective knowledge or to discourses that might enlighten you as to underlying beliefs, opinions, and attitudes about a phenomenon. Increasingly, qualitative health researchers are discovering that there is much to be gained from using inductive analytic techniques on data sets that are generated through different means than simply interviewing or observation. Documents, including such things as policy documents, records of important meetings, lay autobiographical accounts, or public media, may tell us a lot about certain experiential health phenomena if carefully and thoughtfully analyzed (Hodder, 1994). They tend to have the advantage of minimizing the extent to which researchers have shaped their construction (which is of course an important consideration in all of the other data sources I have mentioned), and they can offer us a range of subjective and objective knowledge. Of course, one needs to know what went into the making of a document in order to understand the use to which it ought to be put, and so all documentary sources will be seen to have their limits (lay autobiographies tend to be written by people whose experiences were on the extreme end, policy documents tend to have been written in a manner that is unlikely to embarrass or upset health authorities or governments, and so on). But documents as a primary or collateral source of data are often worthy of consideration.

One particular documentary source that is attracting increasing attention in the qualitative health research world is pre-existing data sets derived from one's own qualitative projects or those of others (Heaton, 2004; Hinds, Vogel, & Clarke-Steffen, 1997; Thorne, 1994). Because data collection using interviews or observations requires a relatively exhaustive effort, many researchers are eager to capitalize on getting full value from the data sets that have already been collected. Those persons who gave of their time to "tell their story" tend to be delighted the more people actually listen, and most researchers are well aware that their primary analysis can only have captured part of the entire context of what they were studying. Secondary analysis can also bring together data sets generated by different researchers on a similar topic, thereby providing a way to reconcile some of the limitations that can come from reliance on the researcher as instrument. However, while secondary analysis can seem appealing in that it allows one to sidestep the time-consuming process of "fieldwork," it requires a very serious and thoughtful treatment of the nature and limitations of the existing data sets, and therefore should not be taken lightly as a way of doing easy "armchair" research.

An exciting development within the qualitative health research field is the introduction of visual representations through the magic of modern technologies. Increasingly researchers are finding that videotaped data offer a much different approach to studying behavioral patterns, for example, in a manner that reduces the problematic influence that a participant observer will necessarily have on the behaviors being observed (Bottorff, 1994). While such strategies don't directly access subjective experience, they are often augmented by other techniques, in some cases building analysis and interpretation of what is captured electronically or on film into the research encounters with patients.

Although each of these sources can and will be used in a primary sense, there is also considerable value in tapping their potential as collateral data sources for a study whose data derive from other sources.

TEXT BOX 4.1

Learning Complexity

To better understand how self-care decision-making is learned and enacted by persons affected by chronic disease, Thorne and colleagues conducted a secondary analysis using interpretive description with data sets from two prior studies involving interviews and think-aloud recordings by persons with chronic illnesses in relation to their self-care decision-making processes. Comparing across contexts and data collection approaches, they learned that taking control of self-care management reflected a conscious decision to attend to the specific manifestations of the illness and to manage social context, lifestyle, and health care. On the basis of this analysis, they documented patterns in the strategic choices patients made in interpreting expert advice and biomarkers, creating individualized standards, and theorizing complexity. The findings from this kind of analysis compel us to reframe conventional understandings of what self-care decision making involves for these individuals, shifting our perspective beyond compliance with medical advice and toward a profound respect for the complexity of the challenge.

Thorne, S., Paterson, B., & Russell, C. (2003). The structure of everyday self-care decision making in chronic illness. *Qualitative Health Research, 13*(10), 1337–1352.

In this way, they can help counterbalance the known limitations of the data source and provide at least one additional angle of vision to correct any refractive error that may result from the design decisions. Using alternative data sources as a collateral approach does not, in my opinion, require that you build separate methodological arguments for how you will analyze each form of data separately, but does require some thoughtfulness in advance about the way in which perspectives from one angle will be used to inform the other to create a more transparent audit trail for the eventual analysis.

Finally, a note about the "thoughtful clinician," which I see as a potential "collateral" data source that is quite often neglected in qualitative health research designs. In studies in which the focus is explicitly to challenge what are understood to be deeply held biases within professional health care, one would not likely turn to clinicians for inspiration. However, most qualitative studies are more about systematically harvesting shared and patterned experiential knowledge so that it can be of use in sensitizing or informing the people who are providing care. In such instances, there is in my opinion a tremendous collateral role for the expert practitioner, whose perspective will have been formulated on the basis of having seen many "cases" over time, and who may well be able to spot potential variations and diversities that are beyond the reach of most qualitative studies. For example, if you interview ten people about a phenomenon, it can seem quite convincing if they all see it in much the same way. However, testing that observation against a thoughtful, experienced clinician—selected specifically for that capacity to consider clinical phenomena across time and context—you may learn that this dominant view is linked with a particular clinical setting, demographic group, or care philosophy. The "thoughtful clinician test," built into the design of your qualitative study, may help you avoid some of the analytic errors that the limits of your design pose and thereby create findings that have impact beyond sitting on a shelf. Because you will use the thoughtful clinician perspective with as much critical reflection as you would any other form of data, something doesn't have to be true just because clinicians think it is, but triangulating what the best of them may have observed with what patients tell you they experience can make for a fairly powerful set of findings.

As an aside, I have long been fascinated by how polarized the qualitative health research community has been in privileging patient perspectives over those of professionals as if professionals were, inherently, problematically biased. While those who have personal subjective experience of a phenomenon can add greatly to our understanding, I also think that the subset of informed, thoughtful, expert clinicians can become a wonderful resource for capturing the hard-earned insights that each will have achieved and which may not have been shared collectively or documented in the literature. My own experience, several years ago, tapping the expert knowledge of pediatric clinical nurse specialists with particular expertise in children requiring gastrostomy (direct feeding through a surgical opening to the stomach) convinced me that the experiential knowledge that these clinicians offered was a marvelous source of insight about clinical patterns and themes that would not have been accessible through other available data sources. The findings from that study ultimately did far more to produce knowledge that could sensitize clinicians to the traumatizing subjective experience of the mothers of these children than could patient or caregiver data alone (Thorne, Radford, & McCormick, 1997). From that experience, I find that including a mechanism for locating and tapping the wisdom of those whose professional commitment embeds them in the field every day is often a valuable design element.

Using Multiple Data Sources

As has become apparent in the description of each of these data sources, no one data source is inherently preferable across all studies. Each has its strengths and limitations, and the idea is to match what it is you want to study with the data source(s) that are most likely to produce meaningful answers. If you are able to work with multiple data sources simultaneously, you will reduce the likelihood of falling into the epistemological traps that each of these data sources might set for you. However, since many smaller qualitative health research studies begin at the exploratory stage and are limited by time and resources, single data source studies do play a role. The key to success, however, is developing genuine understanding of what your data source implies and ensuring that you keep the limits of that source front and center in your thinking when it comes time to analyzing and drawing conclusions about your findings.

Strategizing a Credible Study

Following upon the logic of the philosophical underpinnings under which you are operating, and having worked out some basic elements of design, you are ready to expand on the "bare bones" of your interpretive description proposal with some more concrete and explicit decisions relating to such matters as sampling, general data collection and analysis options, and the manner in which you will build into your design those elements that will ensure the credibility of your final product. If you are a newer researcher, you'll find that these decisions are quite challenging, since each of them does have significant implications, few of which will be fully apparent to you until you have run up against them in the field. However, we all had to learn once, and if you do have access to mentors and guides who have gone through all of the steps of a study before, you can minimize the overwhelming feeling of panic that is fairly common in these early conceptual stages.

In some academic disciplines and branches of science, the research proposal will be a relatively straightforward part of the project, because there are clearly established methods that you are expected to follow. With interpretive description, as with most qualitatively oriented projects, it is quite the opposite, and a lot of hard conceptual and intellectual work goes into the early planning stages. However, you can comfort yourself with the knowledge that all of this planning work directly informs the actual doing of the research, and that it is inevitably time well spent. So this is not a stage to rush through, and if you do it well, once you are actually out in the field, you will find that you have already come a long way toward completion.

Sampling

Having ascertained the source(s) that will be best suited to the kind of study you are planning and the kinds of findings you are hoping to be able to generate, you will next need to consider what subset of the theoretical whole "population" you intend to engage with and how you will locate and involve that "sample." In most instances, you are not going to have access to the full complement of people who have encountered a particular phenomenon, and so you'll need to be thinking about what angle of that phenomenon or what representation of that perspective you'll be looking for. Matters of understanding representation, working out sample size, and deciding on sampling procedures are an inherent part of all research plans.

Representation

The notion of representation is a tricky and complex one, and it is best to understand from the outset that your study will not actually "represent" anything other than what it is. The concept derives from the quantitative requirement to produce a mathematical assessment of the probability that the data sources and points of data collection you have used reflect a commonly accepted measure of the whole. Because that form of science is driven by the basic assumption that a "truth" is there to be found, the rule structures around how you make claims in this regard have become quite explicit.

In the qualitative research world, representation is much more akin to the messy and complex business of how we sort out whose voices have been listened to in making societal or political choices. We know all about interest groups, about silent majorities, and about the ubiquitous influence of power, but we still cannot really determine how to make public choices in a manner that is completely true to the philosophical values underlying a concept like "democracy." Similarly, in the research world, we must assume that every voice that we will encounter in trying to expand knowledge about a human experience will have an explicit interest or bias to bring to our attention. Thus, we need to find ways of thinking about the sample subsets we create for the purpose of answering any research question, come up with rational arguments about why they are worth attending to, and estimate what angle of opinion or perspective they are likely privileging or silencing.

Representation is rarely achieved by the mere fact of numbers, since there is no common basis upon which we could agree what the appropriate denominator ought to be. Qualitative researchers would do well to recall Popper's challenge to "naïve induction" expressed as questioning how many thousands of white swans would you have to see before you could safely conclude that there are no black ones (Popper, 1972). Similarly, we can't achieve it by virtue of social hierarchy, since those who claim to speak for the masses (such as leaders of patient advocacy groups) are inherently in positions in which they have distinguished themselves from the masses they purport to represent. Not that they won't have an important story to tell, but it is quite likely to differ from the story that would be told by most of the individuals whose interests they are advancing.

I think we do much better if we understand that representation serves us best as one of those broad social ideals (like dignity or integrity) that is worth keeping in mind, but not technically achievable. This stance forces us to assume that whatever sample we come up with will not in any meaningful way be "representative," but will rather reflect a certain kind of perspective built from an auditable set of angles of vision whose nature and boundaries we can acknowledge and address. The way we come to understand the nature of our samples, the limitations that are inherent in any sampling procedure, and the implications these have for how we think about the findings we eventually generate on the basis of those samples is what will shape the integrity and credibility of our final product. Thus, there is no fundamentally right way to sample, but rather an essential requirement that we conduct our study on the basis of some transparent sampling logic and report on our findings in keeping with what we understand our sample to represent.

Sampling Approaches

Convenience Sampling Most qualitative research relies upon some variation on the theme of "purposive" or "theoretical" sampling to identify which people or situations will become the central focus of the study (Kuzel, 1999; Morse, 1989b; Sandelowski, 1995b). In some instances, a sample created entirely by "convenience" is quite appropriate, in that the group of people who are closest at hand may well be an excellent source of insight for applied qualitative researchers about a phenomenon, particularly in the earliest stages of describing aspects of its shared experience. However, most such groups will reflect commonalities whose features might well skew the researcher's perceptions about the phenomenon and limit his or her credibility in venturing into any interpretation beyond the specific study context. For example, if a study recruits all patients in a particular hospital unit with a particular condition over a one-week period, then the researcher will be obliged to carefully reflect on how those patients might have been similar to or different from the annual patterns within that hospital or in other hospitals in other settings. In this instance, careful attention must be paid to any peculiarities of this context that might render this group of people quite different from the more general population of such patients. If the unit has a particularly charismatic staff complement, a specialized research program, or even exceptional patient "hospitality" services, one can quickly see how shared and common experiences might tell us far more about the experience of the health care setting than about the experience of the clinical population. So, while it isn't wrong to study convenient samples, the basis upon which those samples are presumed to tell us anything beyond the local context will have to be argued through other means. A researcher might, for example, capitalize on a broader literature to depict this particular setting within the larger context, and, in interpreting findings, explicitly critique the possibilities that this sample varies significantly from others. As a general rule, however, while convenient samples can create a strong basis for "description," they tend to create proportionately greater challenges to justifying "interpretation."

Purposive Sampling A somewhat more representative sampling technique is "purposive" or "phenomenal" sampling, in which the settings and specific individuals within them are recruited by virtue of some angle of the experience that they might help us better understand. It is difficult to discuss this technique without using the term "representation," but avoiding that language if at all possible in framing our research intent can be helpful in keeping us honest. For example, using purposive sampling, we might conclude that if we only included female participants in our study sample for a particular condition that affects both men and women, we might misunderstand some important aspects of the experiential accounts that are specific to gender. Often, these most probable variables that are likely to shape health and illness experience can be predicted in advance, and we can generate a list of those about which we'd like to ensure sufficient diversity. The literature can be a particular source of guidance in this matter, since where there is a body of literature that claims differentiation on the basis of one feature or another, we can be certain our critics will challenge us on that basis when we try to present our findings. So the strategy of purposive sampling is to try to identify, in advance of the study, the main groupings or conditions that you will want to have ensured you include in your study so that the eventual findings you produce have the potential of ringing true or seeming reasonable to your intended audience.

A particular and important form of purposive sampling is the strategic identification of "key informants," such as have long been the hallmark of ethnographic studies. The rationale for key informants is that some members of a community will be better equipped than others to provide you with access to what is happening and why it is happening. In the tribal context of early anthropological studies, for example, one might specifically seek out a chief or someone whose societal role afforded a relatively informed perspective on the society as a whole. Another feature of the key informant was willingness to engage in informing the researcher, and, therefore, building strong interpersonal relationships with key informants was a central component of the process of "entering the field." In the health research context, however, one is a little less likely to be able to identify community members with sufficient stature or position to speak for a group in quite the same manner. However, the underlying idea of the key informant might cause you to seek out individuals with extended experiential background or who would have had exposure to groups of people with backgrounds similar to their own, although it would be unlikely that you could identify those you would consider key in relationship to the group in quite the same manner. Unlike the phenomenological context, in which your ideal coresearchers would be willing to share "pure" experience without the benefit of contaminating it with theorizing, the ideal informants for an interpretive description study might well be those "everyday philosophers" (Gubrium, 1988) within the population who had a particular affinity for observing and thinking about the situations within which they found themselves rather than simply living them.

Theoretical Sampling A third main form of sampling that plays a prominent role in interpretive description is theoretical sampling. This term derives from grounded theory methodology (Glaser & Strauss, 1967; Strauss & Corbin, 1998), where it explicitly builds the sampling strategy from the evolving theoretical variations that derive from the data as the study is being conducted. An important element of theoretical sampling is the idea of maximal variation, in that, as hunches about patterns and themes begin to emerge from the initial phases of data collection and analysis, you will need to search out specific types of "cases" in order to know whether what you are seeing so far is anomalous or an artifact of some unexplained characteristics of your current sample or study design. So, for example, if all of your initial study participants report a similar level of emotional discomfort as central to their experience with a particular diagnostic procedure you are studying, you will want to be sure you explicitly search out contrary cases of individuals for whom there was little or no emotional impact. In this way, you refine the phenomenal or demographic variables upon which you are trying to find maximal variation by adding in variables that would not have been apparent before you entered the study. Later in the study, the idea of theoretical sampling takes on a more explicit purpose in fleshing out the groupings or categories of phenomena that you are considering reporting as findings. If you believe, for example, that you have observed three distinct styles of emotional coping as approaches to dealing with the noxious diagnostic procedure, you might use theoretical sampling for further cases within each of the styles to help refine your claims about what differentiates them from one another and what variations occur within them. Further, before drawing premature conclusions that these three styles represented the field, you might, in consultation with your clinical experts, try to uncover cases that did not appear to fit any of these patterns.

Because your intent is uncovering knowledge that may be relevant for clinical practice and not formal theorizing, interpretive description studies do not require the full scale of analytic depth that theoretical sampling contributes in grounded theory methodology. Nevertheless, the principle of reserving some of these sample selection criteria until the data collection is underway, generating them from and in support of the evolving data analysis and interpretation, and explicitly seeking maximal variation on relevant phenomena that seem central to the focus of the study are all well worth building into a design. While theoretical sampling necessarily requires that you reserve some decisions as inherently emergent within the design, and not all ethical review or granting bodies will be entirely comfortable with the idea of a design in which all elements cannot be ascertained in advance, a thoughtful consideration of the principles and the manner in which you would intend to apply them can elegantly and convincingly be made explicit in a good interpretive description proposal.

Finding Terminology to Refer to Sample Members

Another aspect to remember here is that the terminology by which you refer to the people who end up in your study does reveal something about the philosophical position that you are taking in your research and the claims you are making about their role within the research process. The term "informant" has a long history within ethnographic circles, and reflects those individuals within a culture or society identified as being particularly familiar with the relevant elements of the culture and who were willing to spend the time to explain them to you. Needless to say, the quality of a study is quite dependent upon the key informant selection, since, if you emphasized the perspective of a community member with an axe to grind, you could jeopardize the integrity of your entire interpretive description project. Further, because many communities are made up of distinct "factions," and your key informant choices could be well known, you might well find that certain perspectives within the community could become lost to you while others are privileged. So the idea of tapping "experiential experts" was a central one, but not without its challenges. In the current context, many qualitative health researchers avoid the use of the term "informant" because they believe it distances them from the phenomenon of interest, and perhaps also because it may seem to have a somewhat sinister connotation within the public context. They similarly avoid the term "subject" because it seems to objectify and compartmentalize the human beings with whom they are hoping to have a more full and engaged interaction. However, where you are simply observing and not actively engaging with people, such as in some grounded theory studies, the term "subject" may still have some value.

Within some qualitative research traditions, the term "co-researcher" has emerged as one alternative terminological possibility. This term implies, however, that there is something of an equal partnership between the researcher and the individual being studied, with comparable motivations for the nature and quality of the research product. In a phenomenological study in which a researcher and an individual commit to an extensive engagement of sequenced conversations to systematically uncover layers of meaning inherent in a particular subjectivity that is of concern to them both, the term "co-researcher" may well be an accurate expression. Similarly, in participatory action research in which the researcher has been engaged by a group in its effort to surface its embedded knowledge as a source of power to mobilize change, the term would reflect that distinctive balance of roles. However, in much of what we currently read within the qualitative health research domain, the use of the term "co-researcher" seems to reflect a "feel good" self-congratulatory statement rather than any meaningful procedural commitment. Worse, it seems to absolve the scholar of full responsibility for the research product, despite the likelihood that the subject of the scholar's attention is unlikely to be awarded co-authorship or substantive credit in the final analysis. In my view, it is a term best reserved for those rarer occasions when there is a genuine and ongoing partnership between the knower and the known that shapes all elements of the design, implementation, and ownership of the project.

In this context, then, there are not many good terminological options available for describing the subject of interpretive description research. Because of this, the term "study participant" has become somewhat standard in that it is relatively neutral in its implications and does not carry the implicit unintended baggage from other qualitative research traditions.

Projecting a Sample Size

Interpretive description can be conducted on samples of almost any size. As Patton points out, "Qualitative inquiry seems to work best for people with a high tolerance for ambiguity" (Patton, 2002, p. 242), and the matter of sample size is a case in point. Although the vast majority of studies within this approach are likely to be relatively small (including, perhaps, between 5 and 30 participants), the principles can be applied for various reasons to studies whose sample sizes are much smaller (such as single-case studies) or larger. In my own research, I have used sample sizes as large as 200 in recognition of the complexity of the issues of concern and my understanding of the values and beliefs characteristic of the particular audiences to which I plan to direct my findings.

The best way to justify a sample size is to generate a rationale that is consistent with the research question. How many instances of a thing would we need to include in our observations and analysis in order for the findings to have any merit to those for whom we are conducting the research? If the background literature and disciplinary wisdom suggests that a certain phenomenon occurs commonly within clinical populations and what is needed is a more in-depth exploration of its underlying subjective experiential nature, then we can likely determine that engaging with a small number of individuals experientially familiar with it and willing to share that with us will produce something worth documenting. For example, a nurse researcher seeking to better understand what late-stage cancer patients experience during episodes of shortness of breath so that such individuals might be better supported within the palliative care context might find that the most appropriate study would involve a small available group of individuals carefully selected with clinical staff by virtue of having episodes of that experience, not being in sufficient distress to preclude the appropriateness of interviewing, and having an interest in spending time with the researcher to explain that experience. Elements of recruiting, sample selection, and data collection strategy in this kind of study might be strongly shaped not by formal methodological requirements, but by the most clinically appropriate way to gain access to knowledge about what it feels like to become breathless toward the end of life. In using this somewhat extreme example of a clinical study, I illustrate that interpretive description has become a frame for following a disciplinary logic as to

- what knowledge we need,
- what options there are for getting as close to it as we reasonably can, and
- how we can enact that inquiry in a manner that is most respectful and consistent with both ethical research guidelines and the foundations of ethical clinical practice.

In the above example, it would be relatively easy to understand why a small sample, handled carefully, might produce the knowledge we are seeking. However, there will be many other kinds of clinical studies in which an overly small sample is likely to do an injustice to the topic and lead us into the kind of illogic that "naïve induction" implies (Sandelowski, 1995b). Unfortunately, in trying to be helpful to researchers and give them a published basis for defending small studies, certain authors, such as Morse (1989b), who estimated that six might be a reasonable sample in a phenomenological study, or Kuzel (1999), who suggested that five to eight participants might be sufficient for a homogenous group, have inadvertently found themselves cited as justification for the inherent value of small samples. In some instances, these citations reflect a hollow defense for sample sizes that would ultimately minimize a study's chance of attaining sufficient depth to allow for reporting beyond "thin" description or making any meaningful contribution to the field. While small studies are the way in which most of us learn qualitative technique, and many smaller studies have in fact generated highly respected original findings, the trend toward a rapid proliferation of very small studies has not served the overall field of qualitative health research to best advantage, and has in fact compromised the acceptance of qualitative findings outside of the methodological community.

Setting Limits

Because there is no firm and fast rule regarding what constitutes the right sample size for an interpretive description study, it is incumbent upon the researcher to generate a coherent and defensible claim about the proposed number of cases, subjects, or instances that would have to be included in the study in order for its results to be worthwhile. In my experience, a proposal can most effectively communicate the researcher's intention by providing both a range and an explanation for why the upper and lower limits have been selected. Typically, the lower number might be that of the fewest instances which you'd consider you need to understand in order to be able to discern what constituted common aspects across them. I often tell my students an early lesson I had in this regard during my initial foray into qualitative research when six of the eight families I interviewed had surnames starting with the same letter of the alphabet. While initials are unlikely to be an overly meaningful variable in the lives of families experiencing cancer, had the sample revealed such an extraordinarily dominant variable relating to family dynamics, for example, I might easily have misread its relevance with the analysis and over-inscribed it with some powerful interpretive meaning. This early lesson taught me never to assume that what seems most evident across cases in smaller studies is necessarily the relevant finding.

It is not uncommon or inappropriate for time and resources to become a reasonable element in the decision to constrain sampling within an interpretive description study. Few of us within the health field have unlimited access to both, and we know that grant funding and ethical approval involve arbitrary boundaries on a discrete project. Nevertheless, if these become the primary rationale for setting the study limits, the logic of qualitative science is disserved. My recommendation would be to take these into consideration in the selection of study scope and intent and to ensure, if the study is to be smaller, that you have articulated the kind of problem that can reasonably be tackled with the anticipated exposure. To believe that you can generate coherent, integrated new theory about a clinical phenomenon on the basis of having interviewed a half dozen conveniently recruited informants is to completely misunderstand how useful qualitatively derived knowledge is constructed and evaluated. However, offering a meaningful clinical description, framed in such a manner that it raises the questions and concerns that a disciplinary lens can bring to bear on a complex problem, may be an entirely worthy objective for a smaller study.

Because there is no objective justification for the specific number of people, cases, or instances that are required in order to conduct an interpretive description, you do need to consider how you can justify an appropriate stopping point. Some researchers estimate an upper limit on the cases they will include in their studies and reasonably conclude that, when they enter the field, they can adjust their scope according to the nature of the study within those limits. Certainly, if some of the people that you interview turn out to be poor informants, or your exposure to them is much less intensive or in-depth than you might have wished, you are likely to want to expand your numbers. Or, if the sample you have acquired has given you a glimpse into a theoretical variable that may be quite relevant but you haven't included in your sample, you may need to expand your data collection in order to generate an interpretive analysis that is built upon data rather than imagination.

However, the more common experience of field researchers is to recognize, on entering any clinical field, that the phenomenon of interest is in fact far more interesting and complicated than they had initially anticipated. Human stories tend to provide you with tantalizing "distractors," many of which could be clues to important new aspects, but you won't know immediately which would lead you into blind alleys and which might ultimately be productive lines of inquiry. Depending on the fundamental makeup of their character and the situation in which they find themselves (such as time pressure to complete a degree), individual researchers will operate on the basis of quite different instincts. The instinct for some researchers is to narrow the focus and try to put blinders on to obscure anything in the field that does not seem directly pertinent to the question at hand. This kind of researcher is looking for an excuse to get out of the field quickly before too much data confuses his or her analysis. The other extreme is the researcher who will always have more questions and curiosities, and perpetually assume that the key to unlocking the entire conceptualization will be the gathering of just a little bit more data. The kind of assistance that a methodological orientation ought to provide, then, is not an explicit justification, but rather a nudge to consider which kind of situation you are in and create a logic that ensures a balance.

An unfortunate (in my opinion) pattern in much qualitative health research within the applied disciplines in the current climate is an overreliance on the notion of *saturation* as a justification for leaving the field and concluding data analysis. While it neatly fits within a research proposal and sounds reasonable to the uninformed ear, it is important to understand that the idea of saturation, whether data or theoretical, is entirely and inherently dependent upon the coherence of the argument that you are building. In keeping with the sociological origins of grounded theory, the standard of theoretical saturation becomes a basis for judging the quality of specific pieces of scholarship because it implies that the researcher has pursued the variance required to make certain theoretical claims about the full range of configurations within the basic social process behavior. In that context, the claim of theoretical saturation (or, for that matter, its cousin "redundancy") is one that expresses confidence that no new variations on the theory will emerge from additional data collection. While I have great respect for those who use this concept in the context of actual theory building, I find it highly problematic as a loosely used construct to justify that one has obtained sufficient data to fully understand all that is potentially relevant about the clinical phenomenon in question. In the applied health disciplines, it is inherent in the practice mandate that patients theoretically represent infinite variation in relation to their experiences with health care. Thus, in the disciplinary context of health research, the idea that one can claim that no new variation could emerge seems antithetical to the epistemological foundations of practice knowledge. Instead, a more honest assessment of what one is able to discern on the basis of what one has had exposure to seems more consistent with the kind of clinical reasoning logic that will reach the intended audience.

For that reason, it seems fair to suggest that smaller interpretive description studies are justified in having set somewhat arbitrary sample limits, as long as they show recognition that there would always be more to study, and larger studies can defend their expanded scope on the basis of the kind of relevant variation and complexity that their burning question entails at this juncture in our evolution toward answering it.

Thinking Through Data Collection and Analysis

Your research proposal will necessarily go beyond claims of what data and how much you will seek, and there is much to be said about the conduct of data collection and analysis. A more in-depth discussion on these processes in action is the focus of later chapters in this book. At the initial proposal-writing stage, however, it is important to be able to comment intelligently on what rules and principles you intend to follow in gathering and making sense of data, and to project ahead to the kinds of analytic steps you will take to produce findings. For example, it is difficult to imagine an interpretive description study that does not include some elements of *concurrent data collection and analysis*, and that the analytic process that the disciplinary interpretive mind will bring to that aspect of the research would not involve *constant comparative analysis*. These two ideas are fairly central to a way of studying phenomena in which you start with the assumption that aspects of the reality that you are studying are socially constructed and that to uncover knowledge about them you will compare and contrast different kinds of manifestations of them. While straight description could occur in a study that gathers data first and thinks later, interpretive description will inevitably require that the ongoing engagement with data be strategically employed to confirm, test, explore, and expand on the conceptualizations that begin to form as soon as you enter the field.

Another central element of data collection and analysis in interpretive description is that you are seeking the kind of knowledge that must be inductively generated from within the data, and developed within the context of that data. So, ideas (frameworks, theories) that you bring into the study will have to be carefully noted and regularly examined to be sure that they are not influencing what you see and hear in ways that you don't intend. While that precaution can be relatively easy to take with an explicit theory that is compartmentalized in your mind, it is a little more difficult to do that with clinical or disciplinary knowledge (as in the old adage that it would not have been a fish that discovered water) (Schein, 1987). For example, in studying self-care decision making among persons with a chronic disease, you may find it difficult to "turn off" the part of your clinical mind that immediately wants to embark on patient teaching when your study participant begins to explain his or her intricate rationale for manipulating treatment protocols. Some careful thought as to the manner in which you will deal with your known disciplinary preconceptions—and you will distinguish those that may be socially constructed as opposed to fundamental (the inherent dignity of all persons, for example)—will help you create a personal guide to staying on the research path once you enter the clinical field for the purpose of inquiry (Robinson & Thorne, 1988).

Because research proposal formats typically require a clear separation between data collection and analysis, you will be looking for ways of summarizing what you propose to do in the field in a manner that does justice to the underpinnings of the method but also helps those less familiar with qualitative approaches in general (or interpretive description in particular) feel comfortable that there is indeed a design logic. In an earlier era, some qualitative researchers were inclined to describe the processes of data collection and analysis in somewhat soft and fuzzy language (with analysis being a form of "magic," or findings "emerging from the data," for example) (May, 1994; Morse, 1994b). Although these are useful experiential observations (indeed the workings of the human mind truly are quite marvelous and fascinating), they tend not to serve the demands of those seeking to explain their study approaches to unimaginative audiences. For this reason, it becomes important to identify the main approaches that will be employed and the sequence within which they will be used in concrete and explicit language within your proposal.

Depending on the data source(s) you have selected, you will find excellent resources within the qualitative research literature to guide your process. It is a good idea, for example, to understand something of group dynamics and to build a skill set for communicating with groups before you try to enact a focus group study. Similarly, there is a great deal to be learned about research interviewing beyond what you may already know from the clinical interview context if interviewing is to become your primary data collection strategy. In fact, if you are proficient in interviewing patients for the purpose of assessment and taking clinical histories, for example, you may find that a lot of painful unlearning is required before you enter the research arena to ensure that you aren't falling back on old patterns of "leading the witness." Similarly, participant observation requires a particular mindset and collection of reflective self-checking skills in order to tease out what is happening to you personally from what it is that you are seeing. So some specific learning in relation to the specific data source is always a good idea.

While the qualitative research world is full of "cookbooks" that break out the processes of data collection and analysis into simple and neatly sequenced intellectual operations, the actual business of data collection and analysis is considerably more complex (Morse, 1994c). However, a vague or overly complex statement of what these processes will look like may not be an advantage to your interpretive description research proposal. My recommendation, therefore, is to draw upon these kinds of guidelines, where they seem appropriate, as a general statement of what you expect to occur. For example, a number of authors (e.g. Colaizzi, 1978; Giorgi, 1985; Strauss & Corbin, 1998) have included in their methodological guidelines an abbreviated sequenced set of steps that many researchers find helpful to draw upon. However, unlike cookbooks, they tend to work far better as general conceptual guides than rulebooks, and recognizing from the outset that you'll be "informed" by them rather than "doing" them will help you write your plan with integrity.

Building In Credibility Indicators

In the proposal stage of an interpretive description, you will also be required to say something about the plan you intend for ensuring that your research results have some integrity. It is fair to say that the matter of quality within qualitative health research is a highly complex and challenging topic, with much still unresolved and many ongoing disputes on the table. However, a research proposal is incomplete without some demonstration that the worth of the final product of research is not based simply on the researcher's claims (Thorne & Darbyshire, 2005) and that certain steps and procedures within the process of the research will be undertaken to ensure that there is a quality to the ingredients and to the outcome.

The validity and reliability that we are familiar with in the quantitative research world do not match the specific philosophical assumptions and aims that underscore qualitative work (Leininger, 1994; Thorne, 1997). However, general principles do have meaning in the sense that qualitative researchers agree that it is important to have quality criteria reflecting agreed-upon ideas about the bases upon which data have been generated and analyzed and conclusions rendered. We recognize that the claims made about a health phenomenon by a researcher within the current sociopolitical context have a different currency than would similar claims made by an informed bystander, a journalist, or a politician. A significant measure of that privilege comes from the assumption that the claims extend far beyond mere "opinion," and in fact are based on recognizable ways of empirical reasoning. This platform of expertise that scientists benefit from would erode rapidly in the absence of shared bases for determining the worth of research. In the qualitative research world, despite the ongoing and lively debate as to how best accomplish credibility in our research designs, the researcher is obliged to show serious thoughtfulness to this challenge and to identify some appropriate techniques that will be employed to assure the integrity of the process and product.

In the context of clinical qualitative health research, we might take that set of obligations one step further, and recognize that our species of new knowledge will be written up in a form that enlightens our intended clinical audience about dimensions of the thing we are studying, and consequently that our findings may be taken up in the practice context without the benefit of what other scientists might consider essential testing. For example, if our in-depth interviews with cancer patients reveal a common preference for certain ways of expressing compassion, clinicians reading a report might find themselves unconsciously adjusting their behaviors in practice. While we can generally assume that formal clinical procedural change will require systematic review of evidence, there is much within the clinical world that is highly sensitive to the findings of a well-timed, articulate, and powerful qualitative research presentation, especially if it matches the "clinical instincts" that our audiences are already predisposed to favor. Because so much of what we study qualitatively has the potential to tug at heartstrings or feed biases, there is considerable risk in uncritically accepting the findings of any individual study.

While credibility can be enhanced by application of a wide range of procedures, some of those that have been particularly well received within the qualitative health research community are those articulated by Leininger (1994), who conceptualized the six distinct evaluative criteria that should be considered as credibility, confirmability, meaning-in-context, recurrent patterning, saturation, and transferability, and the "trustworthiness" elements of credibility, transferability, dependability, and confirmability used by Lincoln and Guba to position a study as "worth paying attention to" (1985, p. 290). Within each of these dimensions, various researchers draw upon specific techniques that they intend to apply, such as triangulation of data sources to enhance credibility, "member checking" to test confirmability, or expert panel analysis to support claims of dependability. While these techniques may bolster confidence in some dimension of credibility, the specific approaches that a researcher selects should be generated on the basis of what he or she is attempting to achieve beyond methodological precision or technical accuracy. Later, in Chapter 13, I will elaborate on what I consider better ways to think about the objective of credibility procedures within interpretive description, orienting our choices toward such criteria as epistemological integrity, representative credibility, analytic logic, and interpretive authority. In order that interpretive description products actually contribute to disciplinary knowledge, I suggest that it is important for applied health researchers to position their inquiries in relation to an additional set of ideal criteria, including moral defensibility, disciplinary relevance, pragmatic obligation, contextual awareness, and probable truth (Thorne, 1997).

All of these credibility measures orient us to the requirement that we build in sufficient strategies to keep our evolving data collection and analysis on target with our ultimate research purpose. They create a means by which we can demonstrate to others—both in advance of our study and in the eventual report—a form of "reflexive accounting" designed to lend a measure of validity to the conclusions we reach (Altheide & Johnson, 1994).

Planning and Adapting

The paradox of good qualitative research planning is that you can't fully appreciate what will happen in a study or what protections you might need to include in order to ensure that all of the threats to credibility and trustworthiness will be overcome along the way. While a loose plan (of the "trust me to figure it out as I go" variety) is highly unlikely to pass muster with your graduate supervisory committee or your grant funding review panel, an overly rigid one may lock you into procedures and elements that are unnecessary or even counterproductive. Further, the more complex and intricate your plan is, the harder it can be to assume a standpoint above it and see the "forest for the trees" once you are actually in the middle of the project. Simply writing a logical design and then following it will not ensure high-quality findings, and paying compulsive attention to the design details creates the risk of turning your study into a hollow exercise.

The point of an interpretive description research plan is to create a solid foundation of the principles underlying the choices you are going to be making along the journey, and to articulate a logical and credible sequence of intended intellectual and procedural activities in order to reach your goal. You are, in effect, positioning yourself to be able to engage deeply in understanding the phenomenon that sparked your interest in the first place, to invoking a full set of analytic steps to knowing its structure and nature, and to creating the building blocks upon which you hope to generate meaningful new knowledge. While interpretive description does not give you the (apparent) luxury of a lockstep set of design decisions, it offers a framework within which the design decisions that work for your particular question can be effectively set forth. Although that may initially feel like a somewhat less solid foundation than you might have with a prefabricated design, it has two real advantages: (1) the design you come up with will be one that supports the particular kind of question you are asking, and (2) the planning logic that you put into the initial phases of your study will serve you brilliantly in avoiding multiple pitfalls in the actual conduct of your research. Your goal, after all, is to come away with findings that advance understanding in your field, not simply to have lived through the process!

While it is sensible to make some of the overall design decisions on a somewhat pragmatic basis, the key to your success will lie in your ability to predict and appreciate the implications of each decision for the integrity of the whole. As you explore all of the available options, you realize that you must make trade-offs and limit your choices within the full set of possibilities (Patton, 2002).

In this set of chapters, we've provided a brief overview of the origins of interpretive description and the logic of research project planning. In the next set of chapters, we will delve in more detail into the specific implications, within interpretive description, of some of the many ways of inductively engaging with clinical data.

PART

II

INTERPRETIVE DESCRIPTION
IN PROCESS

CHAPTER SIX

Entering the Field

Having thought through a study proposal, you are ready to move into conversations about the actual process of conducting an interpretive description. As with any design, there can be a gap between the articulation of an idea in the proposal stage and the actual doing once you have clearance to go forward. What can read as a simple line within a proposal (such as "once I have gained entry into the field") can turn out to be a complicated and difficult dynamic once the very real nuances of your particular situation reveal themselves and you are faced with dilemmas for which you may not have been prepared. This again is a time in which colleagues and mentors who have walked the path of research before in your settings can be invaluable, and if you haven't cultivated such colleagues before this stage, this might be the appropriate moment! In this and the following four chapters, I will discuss the kinds of representation and responsibility issues that commonly arise for newer researchers in particular, and will present some thoughts about solutions.

Just as the design logic of interpretive description study permits considerable latitude in relation to most steps within the proposed research, the various dimensions of "interpretive-description-in-action" can be enacted in many different ways by different researchers within their distinctive contexts. What interpretive description provides is a rationale for working out these elements according to the requirements of an applied discipline—that is, a discipline in which action must necessarily occur even in the absence of the new knowledge, but the new knowledge you are seeking has the potential to shape or influence aspects of that action simply by its capacity to shift perception among practitioners. Thus, the choices that one makes with interpretive description draw from the wonderful legacy that the social science methods have left us, but select from them with the full mantle of responsibility that ideas within a practice discipline entail. This principle will guide all aspects of the choices each researcher makes within this rubric, and will distinguish the findings of interpretive descriptions from the products that have adhered more closely to the tenets of the other methods.

That said, the challenge now is to begin to identify what options can be consistent with an interpretive description logic, and how one might work through the decisions with which a research project will necessarily confront one. Here, I'll offer some thoughts and opinions, many of which could be said to be a matter of personal preference and style rather than fundamental requirements of the interpretive description approach. If the reader will indulge me the opportunity to offer the kind of guidance that I might share in discussion with colleagues and graduate students in relation to these challenges, then the ideas here are offered as one basis for guiding sound logic in the interpretive description context, not prescription as to its requirements.

Situating Self Within the Research Role

While armchair theorizing can be quite compelling fun, clinician researchers really come alive when they are finally at the stage of being able to enter the research setting and engage with the sources of data. In most instances, people (study participants) will be the primary source of data, and a fascination for people within the clinical context is most likely what inspired the study in the first place. However, doing research is seldom what one imagined it would be at the outset of a research career, and there are many caveats and cautions related to dealing with people that are well worth attending to in order to prevent problems that can threaten your continuation within the research setting, the integrity of the data you will collect, or potentially the credibility of the entire project. Many of these elements combine ethical, theoretical, and practical aspects, and so discussion of these issues will be intertwined with the description of common challenges and some suggested solutions.

Despite being drawn to qualitative research because of their enthusiasm for subjective experiential clinical knowledge, many clinicians find the transition into the role of researcher considerably more difficult than they had first imagined. One tends to feel confident and comfortable interacting with clients within one's practice setting, and the idea of having the luxury of spending more time with the people who have inspired that enthusiasm is highly attractive. However, there are various aspects of that "former self" that you will have to abandon in order to take on the new challenge of becoming the instrument of credible and meaningful research.

Tracking Reflections

First, as was discussed in Chapter 3, you will need to carefully acknowledge and document the nature and substance of the ideas you hold about the phenomenon you are studying before you enter the field. This process will continue throughout your research process, but perhaps most particularly during the data-collection and analysis processes. While reflexivity is an inherent element of all qualitative inquiry, and reference to it is easily included in any plan, the process, relevance, and meaning of it are far from straightforward (Finlay, 2002). Nevertheless, documenting something of what is happening to you subjectively and conceptually within the research engagement becomes a core element informing your inductive analytic process.

You might accomplish this through a field notebook, or a personal reflective "journal" that will become an important part of your research documentation. In general, although it might seem so self-evident that you would never forget it, it is always best to create explicit places to document such background material, and to ensure that you have access to it for further elaboration as the research unfolds and for later reference. While it may not become "data" per se, it does become a very critical part of what you will need to understand the implications of your own role in data collection and construction. Depending upon your own preference and style, you might maintain a single research notebook (electronic or actual) in which you record all of the thoughts, questions, and ideas that occur to you as your study unfolds. Or you might create separate places in which to record background preconceptions (theoretical allegiances, your expert clinical opinion, other sources of prior knowledge) and your ongoing analytical notes (questions, inspirations, and evolving interpretations). In either case, ensure that these become part of your life as a researcher, that they are always available (for those quick notes in the middle of the night, etc.), and that they are regularly maintained. As with all data, it goes without saying that you will want to ensure you have regular mechanisms for backing these up, or protecting yourself against loss during the project.

Learning Not to Lead

A second aspect of becoming an effective researcher has to do with "undoing" your clinical practice engagement and communication techniques. Most likely, you are accustomed to greeting new clients with the confidence of a seasoned practitioner, to expecting some clarity within the roles (of them seeking assistance and you knowing how to provide it), and to communicating with them, at least initially, on the basis of an explicit or implied set of clinical parameters (the assessment interview, for example). You know the scene, you know where you are going with each conversation, and you are, for the most part, in control of the direction that the interaction will take. While you very likely have engaged in many clinical interactions that seem less purposeful than that which I am describing, those new to the applied research world are almost always surprised at how difficult it really can be to shift into this new persona. Essentially you are taking on the role of someone who does not know, who has entered the study participants' world in order to know, and who cannot bring that expertise into shaping the conversation as it unfolds. Research interviews, as we will see later in this chapter, are markedly different from clinical interviews, and the clinician's tendency to "lead the witness" can take considerable undoing as you work toward mastering the skill of research interviews (Hutchinson & Wilson, 1994; Lipson, 1989). A classic source of excellent guidance on the research interview that has been adopted and applied across a range of methodological traditions is James Spradley's text on the "ethnographic interview" (1979). Through a detailed depiction of the attitude, conversational options, and focus of the interview itself, Spradley's text has helped many clinical researchers become aware of their clinical communication habits and create strategies for managing those that might influence the research interview in an untoward manner.

Disclosing the Discipline

A third issue is how one will introduce or portray oneself to potential study participants. In an earlier chapter, we raised some of the considerations relative to positioning oneself within the study, but that step is quite different from explaining oneself to those with whom one hopes to engage to learn something about subjective experiential matter. For example, if we frontload our introductions to potential study participants with theoretical positions (feminist, critical social theory, humanist, holistic, and so on), we already bias who is likely to accept our invitation to participate and what they will say when we engage with them. Alternatively, if we hold strong theoretical views and attempt to mask them, we are clearly misrepresenting our intent. A potential research participant who believes that we are seeking knowledge to help nurses better understand patients with a particular condition may be much more comfortable accepting our invitation than would one who believes that we are studying people with the condition in order to explore a power imbalance within the care of patients overall. So our motivation does become an important element in shaping our access to data as well as the constructions that we will arrive at on the basis of our engagement with the field.

One particular challenge for health clinician researchers is the recognition that many patients might well relish the opportunity to spend a significant period of time with a health care professional for reasons other than contributing to knowledge. They may unwittingly hope that they'll gain further information about their condition, have the opportunity to confirm their own theories or strategies about managing it, or seek to create a somewhat indebted relationship with an "insider" within the system. Thus, the process of situating oneself does require some careful strategizing in order to avoid inappropriate expectations and ensure as much clarity as possible within the research engagement process. These steps become part of the critical process of setting and maintaining appropriate boundaries within the research relationship (Dickson-Swift, James, Kippen, & Liamputtong, 2006). While acknowledging a professional allegiance does create these kinds of drawbacks, obscuring that information seems quite unethical. Thus, the researcher is required to find a way to explain the interest in the topic from a professional background, combined with the current role of being the "learner" from the individual who holds the expertise in subjective experience—the patient him or herself. This two-dimensional introduction provides some clarity in both the source of interest in the question and in the expectations for engagement, and permits the researcher to make explicit that the benefit of the research will be knowledge that may help enlighten fellow professionals for the benefit of future patients.

Stepping out of Role

Despite all good intentions to be true to the researcher role, I doubt that it is really possible to discard one's larger social mandate as a health care professional engaging in the research of one's profession (Robinson & Thorne, 1988). It is well recognized by clinical researchers that occasions will arise in which the distress of the study participant, the seriousness of his or her misinformation, or the acuity of the clinical concern may have to "trump" the research agenda. One mechanism that has been suggested as a rule of thumb for such situations is to bifurcate the research interview—gather data first, and shift into a clinical conversation afterwards. In my own view, that may not always be feasible or even ethical, and therefore a more conceptual understanding of what is happening in the situation and what will or will not constitute research is required. Here, the value of the reflective notebook comes into play, because it becomes a place where that fine line between being therapeutic and serving a research agenda can be explicitly dissected and examined. Through regular self-inquiry, the researcher can develop a multidimensional understanding of where the "learner side" is dominant and where some elements of the "clinician side" may have been called into action. When the interview has shifted for all or part of a session into the clinical context for any reason, decisions will have to be taken with regard to whether the data have been "tainted" such that they cannot be used within the analysis, or whether elements of the data are still appropriate for research use. Clearly, that decision will depend upon the phenomenon being studied and the interaction between the specific clinical encounter and the story being told.

Revealing and Concealing

A related tricky issue that arises in the context of a number of interpretive description studies is the explicit personal location of the researcher within the content of the question that is being posed. This issue arises most dramatically where the topic is one for which there would be common recognition that personal experience shapes understanding. For example, in a study of interpersonal violence, it might be important for the researcher to develop a clear and consistent message as to his or her own relationship to the topic, not only to frame the interest, but also because he or she is likely to be asked. Since "I don't feel comfortable disclosing that information to you" is quite likely to set up a natural resistance to the interview process, more respectful and constructive options are in order. Most researchers do decide to avoid revealing personal information unless explicitly asked, since "sharing" does add to the burden of keeping a research interview on target for its intended purpose. Where the researcher has personal experience, the study participant is much more likely to assume a shared understanding and therefore disinclined to go into depth on what might be key elements inherent in the phenomenon under study. There is also a great temptation to "compare notes," which then conveys the idea that there is a "right way" to have experienced the matter. It is always important to remember that there are very powerful "social protocols" for sharing discourse at play, and having entered the space of being "fellow travelers" in a challenging world, it can be almost impossible to regain the stance of the "outsider" inquirer.

In my view, there is no inherently right answer to the dilemma of disclosure, particularly in relation to sensitive topics. You may decide to find a way of diverting the study participant's question away from your own experience and back toward his or her own, perhaps even indicating that you would be open to having that conversation following the interview proper. Or you may explain why, in your opinion, it is important that the focus of the interview remain on the study participant, as possibly knowing your own (nonclinical) relationship to the topic could inadvertently influence the way the story is told. Just as with clinical knowledge, emphasizing your enthusiasm for the opportunity to learn from "their" experience rather than assuming that your prior knowledge is valid can be an effective way to sidestep these difficult conversations. However, some study participants will insist, and researchers tend not to want to tell a lie. So thinking through how, if you do have some personal exposure to the issue, you will explain that without undue fanfare and then guide the interview back to the study participant's story, accounting for any potential influence that the disclosure might have on the data that subsequently arise, will be an important element in preparing yourself to conduct the interpretive description.

Negotiating Informed Consent

Although your setting and institution will undoubtedly have explicit procedures and policies related to informed consent to participate in a study, the challenge of attending with integrity to informed consent, both at the outset and on an ongoing basis, has long been recognized as a particular challenge for qualitative researchers in general. Essentially, because the focus of your inquiry is human subjective experiential knowledge, the researcher cannot fully predetermine what will happen in the research encounter. Unlike quantitative investigations, in which the specific questions that will be posed are an essential element in the study design, there is an "emergent" quality to interpretive description (as with many qualitative approaches) that explicitly requires following leads suggested by the study participants and capitalizing on linkages among bits of data as you progress through the research. Because of this, the "interview schedule" characteristic of conventional descriptive research would be a misnomer. Rather, most practitioners of interpretive description navigate the informed consent process with an explanation of the relationship between data collection and analysis combined with some formal indication of their "best guess" as to how the typical interview will proceed. You might generate "sample trigger questions for initial interview" or a "general focus group guide," for example, that illustrates the anticipated range and scope of the inquiry, assuring your review panels, institutional setting authorities, and sometimes even proposed study participants of the "general idea" inherent in your design.

Most of us are not terribly accustomed to having a stranger listen at length to our story or focus with serious intent upon our personal experiences and opinions. The experience of "being heard" is well recognized as a profound one, and this becomes important as we reflect on what our study participants reveal as we guide them ever more deeply into describing elements of their subjective experience. The paradox is that really "good data" often reflect deeply felt and rarely articulated material, and as our study participants come closer to such revelations, our moral obligation toward ongoing negotiation of informed consent is intensified.

While it is easy to recognize that coercing ongoing participation through trickery or manipulation would be highly unethical, qualitative researchers can easily lose sight of the implications of neediness, loneliness, or even the feeling of self-importance that can derive from being "studied." These too can be manipulated to advantage in the search for "good data." Thus, the business of informed consent within the interpretive description approach is best constituted as an ongoing moral obligation, enacted in verbal as well as nonverbal behavior, with the goal of creating the optimal conditions to ensure that the people we study reveal what they are comfortable with and no more. As will be discussed in later chapters, there may be considerable value in the strategy of multiple exposures to a study participant in ensuring that consent remains informed. Where an interview becomes emotional or "secret" information is revealed, for example, the researcher might build in a time delay before continuing on that track, allowing for reflection and reconsideration rather than capitalizing on the immediate impulse. Alternatively, the researcher might step back from the inquiry and create a momentary "pause," noting that the interview has entered difficult territory and inviting the participant to take a moment to reflect on whether he or she wishes to continue. Although the nuances and complexities of engaging with study participants in such a manner as to ensure their ongoing consent are beyond the scope of this brief discussion, these few comments are provided simply to locate the expectations of any interpretive description study within this larger context.

Finding Your Tongue

What most health professionals find when they first engage in qualitative research interviews is an uncomfortable sense of "nakedness" without their usual repertoire of conversational tools. While they can get through their introductory remarks fairly easily, the going gets a bit rougher once they are into the interview proper and trying to encourage people to move in the intended direction without overly directing the interaction. Unlike the clinical encounter, the use of value-laden prompts ("that's good," or "I agree," or even "I understand") are generally forbidden, since they clearly let the participant know that a certain species of data will be well received, and imply the corollary that, if there is opposite data within their own complicated situation, it might not. What qualitative research interviews ask you to do is suspend the idea that you know or understand—to prompt for further clarification or elaboration rather than to signal that you understand completely. Responding in this manner feels counterintuitive to most clinicians, for whom conveying the idea of understanding is fundamental to caring communication. One tends to feel rather silly when limited to "hmm hmm" and "say more," and the urge to assure your study participant that you are not one of those dispassionate health care professionals he or she might be referring to can be almost overpowering.

What becomes necessary, then, is a repertoire of "good questions" that you can draw upon as your interviews progress so that you have options beyond the dispassionate "hmm hmm." Kinds of questions that you may rehearse in advance so that they are ready when you need them might include: "I'm really interested in the way you are describing that. Can you give me a bit more detail about how that happened?" or "Was that surprising to you?" or "A few minutes ago, you mentioned X. Was this new episode anything like that, or did you see some differences?" With these kinds of questions, you are signaling sustained interest in your study participants' thought processes and experiences, encouraging some reflective interpretation, and communicating an interest in the detail of their experience that will in itself express respect and compassion. Within interviews, it is also possible to capitalize on the luxury of learning from your study participants and not compromising your data while at the same time facilitating the flow of the interview. Because you are concurrently collecting and analyzing data, it is entirely appropriate to draw generally on the larger data set as a point of reference, using such questions as "I've heard from some other patients that, just as in your situation, this aspect of the care process seemed most challenging. Have you any thoughts as to why that might be?" or "I've been hearing somewhat similar things from others, and I'd love to better understand it. Can you tell me more?" What helps, when bereft of your usual mechanisms for expressing human kindness and interest in your patients, is a clear understanding that, effectively conducted, your research interview will leave your study participant feeling honored by being listened to deeply, and with the hope that his or her experiential knowledge may contribute to the betterment of care for others in the future. By concluding your interview with a summary of the key themes that you have heard (and will take away and reflect upon), you will have demonstrated the value that the interview has had toward that greater purpose.

Constraining Your Influence

A final priority within the process of situating yourself with your study participants is recognizing and taking responsibility for your privileged capacity to shape the data collected and analyzed as a result of your engagement with the study. There are two general areas of "influence" that the researcher should be mindful of throughout, both to ensure that the research relationship maintains its ethical base and to safeguard the integrity of the findings.

Earlier, we discussed the matter of disclosing one's disciplinary orientation and understanding that it might create some expectations for the research relationship. Another potential effect of the disciplinary role is that it might afford certain advantages in relation to the data that become available through the research process. Nurses, for example, are well aware that their professional background often makes certain species of data more readily available to them than it might be to other researchers. People assume that nurses would be comfortable with details of various bodily functions, for example, that are normally kept more private. I would imagine that bankers are more likely to hear details of someone's financial status and lawyers to hear about their adventures in tax evasion.

In the world of experiential knowledge, there is no way one can study a phenomenon without running the risk of changing it. Merely by attending to selected aspects of an experience or soliciting elaboration on its elements, the researcher may be inadvertently triggering subtle or not-so-subtle shifts in meaning. In recognition of this, the practitioner of interpretive description must be mindful throughout the study of the bases upon which his or her interpretations are formed and the personal or ideational influence that he or she is having upon the data sources. The point here is that simply by being what and who we are, we will have influenced what is revealed to us and the material that we will be using when we construct our accounts of the study. We can't completely avoid this influence, but we can be mindful of it and take steps to ensure that we are as aware as we can possibly be of the way it plays out and the meaning that our study process will have on the eventual product.

The second dimension of influence control is closely associated with the larger principle of informed consent. When individuals have enrolled in our study, they have been provided with certain information about the nature and purpose of the study and the manner in which the findings will be used. While the explanations may have alluded to the idea that aspects of the analysis would be emergent, and developed on the basis of an iterative analysis, there is generally an agreed-upon understanding of the scope and purpose that must be sustained throughout the study. Because the researcher has the potential of exerting influence upon the participants and therefore upon the data, and because ideas may well arise from the data that were not anticipated at the outset, there is an ongoing obligation to align the direction of the study findings with the motivation of the individuals who participated in creating them. Thus, if individuals have consented to be interviewed as to their experience with preoperative teaching for a particular surgical procedure, they will not expect that the study findings will become a condemnation of the surgical technique or the surgeon's personal habits. While they may consistently have revealed common information about those aspects of their story, particularly if the researcher seemed interested, it would be a significant violation of their consent to divert the product of the research toward objectives they might not have sanctioned.

This matter of constraining one's influence is far from straightforward. However, it is an aspect of situating yourself within the research encounter that must be considered and attended to both at the outset and as the investigation unfolds. And as with all of the dimensions that have been listed here, it provides "something to think about" in the conduct of the research rather than an iron-clad rule as to proper procedure.

Situating Self Within the Setting

A second major challenge associated with situating yourself within the setting is the matter of sorting out how to represent yourself and advocate on behalf of your study within the practice setting in which you are conducting your study or recruiting your study participants. Unlike ethnographers, who tend to assume the need to fight their way into the field and spend time establishing relationships once there, clinical researchers often have a misguided optimism about ease of entry and access. Although they know how to "work systems" as professionals, they often find that these same systems are not nearly as friendly to them once they don the researcher hat.

Insiders and Outsiders

Clinical researchers often have the option of doing a study within an actual setting in which they are familiar by virtue of professional experience or locating their study in a similar setting whose members have not worked as closely with them in this context. As with many of the decisions that one takes in the course of an interpretive description study, there are pros and cons associated with either option, and the best approach will result from a consideration of the implications of each within the specific study context. The value of being an "insider" is that you can bypass the early "introductions" stage and you know who holds authority to support your project. There may be various advantages associated with having insider privilege, including more straightforward access to information, consultation, and background contextual information. However, there are also significant disadvantages that may outweigh the benefits (Field, 1989). Insiders often find it more difficult to "step out of role" and may find themselves drawn into clinical activity during times of research engagement. Clients within a setting may find it highly confusing if the same individual assumes different roles at different times, and there is a significantly increased risk of coercion into participation if the connection between the researcher and the clinical team is apparent. Insiders are also far more likely to absorb untested assumptions about how things are done, and study participants knowing that researchers are insiders may well shape their stories accordingly or avoid raising matters that might put the researcher in a compromising position with colleagues. All of these are daunting propositions, requiring careful attention and reflection to ensure that the research process is managed with the utmost integrity.

In contrast, being an "outsider" to the setting tends to bump one up against all of the predictable resistances that clinical settings are famous for—restricting access to information, prioritizing everything above research, selectively sharing knowledge relevant to the study, and so on. It can take time to build relationships with staff when you don't know the leaders, the factions, and the history that make up the internal culture. You are likely to be seen as an intruder, someone who is associated with extra work on the part of the staff, or worse—someone who may have the hidden motivation of exposing poor practices. Since qualitative health researchers are characteristically interested in understanding how the world looks from the patient's perspective, they may be even more prone than quantitative researchers to suspicion and resistance in this regard. This may take the form of complex permissions sequences, competing ethical approval requirements, or contested "ownership" of patients or information. The net effect of that contextual challenge is that the researcher is likely to become highly sensitized to the plight of the patient attempting to navigate that same system, and potentially hostile to the setting itself.

Navigating Access

As all researchers in the current regulatory context are well aware, access to sites of data collection is highly controlled by a set of checks and balances against coercion, misrepresentation, and misuse of information. It is essential that these various procedures and policies be taken very seriously and that the researcher enter the setting well armed with as full an understanding as possible of the current rule structures and requirements.

It is also the case that, despite their theoretical enthusiasm for the value of knowledge generation, most settings find the researcher to be a bit of a nuisance. There are rules to be explained, information provided, and often a requirement that you work through designated individuals to schedule your access to the setting or to potential recruits for the study. It goes without saying that profound respect for the challenge you impose will go a long way to paving the way forward, and your ability to adapt to the changing climate and accommodate to the needs of the setting (as long as they don't compromise your study) will be instrumental in achieving success. Remember that your clinical colleagues are not as immersed as you are in the rules and procedures of research, and so the obligation to do the work of navigation and to ensure that the appropriate people know what you are doing is yours (Punch, 1994). Some important strategies that are applicable across settings include clear communications about when you will and will not be present, and what you will be doing when you are on site; ensuring that the staff have access to the background information about your study, including full contact information in the event that any problems or questions associated with your study arise; and making every effort to respectfully accommodate the staff's needs where yours and theirs collide.

Watching and Doing

Just as study participants may be influenced by the disciplinary background of the investigator, a clinical setting cannot help but be influenced by the professional credibility of the research "visitor." The case of nurses doing research in a hospital setting is perhaps typical of the challenge. Even if one is simply on site to gather names of prospective study participants, it becomes almost impossible to maintain an entirely neutral stance. You instinctively reach out to steer the patient whose wheelchair has got stuck in a door, find someone to help the patient who is calling for assistance, and step in to help lift where a nurse seems to be struggling with an awkward transfer. For this reason, it is somewhat rare for health professional researchers to consider their observations "pure," and more common to describe their intentions in the form of "participant observation." By acknowledging that dual role, they ensure that careful attention will be paid to the manner in which participation might influence or shape that observation.

Being a participant observer, however, demands thoughtful attention to how much participation and of what kind will be appropriate within the context of your study as well as in keeping with the safety and risk management requirements of the institution. For example, nurse researchers might explicitly describe their participation as involving assisting with basic patient care, but not administering medications or treatments. In all such instances, it will be important to have fully assessed and followed the institution's requirements for documentation and tracking, as you have *de facto* become a part of the context that might affect patient outcomes.

Many clinical researchers find that some level of participant observation within an interpretive description study can be a real asset to the project if handled wisely. It is much easier to build trusting relationships with staff (and gatekeepers) if you are helping out rather than sitting like the proverbial bump on a log, and a modicum of participation can help you gain further perspective on the context. It can demonstrate respect for the members of the setting, and give them something in return for their efforts to support you in the study. As with all of these delicate balancing acts, however, it will be of the utmost importance to keep notes and reflect on the implications that the participation may have had on what you have access to, what you see, and how you understand it.

Staying Safe

Although researchers using interpretive description may access their study participants through clinical or similar systems, in many instances they may engage with those individuals in settings or contexts that are distinct from the clinical situation. For example, whereas access to information and the initial introduction to a potential participant may be highly regulated within the clinic, once the individual has accepted the invitation to participate in your study, he or she is unlikely to consider the clinic to have any bearing on the continuation of that relationship. Further, since interpretive description studies commonly take place within the natural context to the extent possible, home visits or conducting interviews at offices or other convenient locations are quite common. While conducting research in this manner does get you out of the way of the regimented environment of the clinic, it raises another important set of challenges.

Health professionals are accustomed to dealing with all manner of individuals, including those that might be considered somewhat unsavory or downright unsafe within the clinical context. They rely upon the "safety nets" that are implied within the health care setting, and typically work hard to overcome any apparent tension that encounters with such "difficult" patients might imply. Thus, for those accustomed to institutional settings, it is quite possible to have an inflated sense of confidence that one can handle any encounter. When the encounter shifts to the setting that may be most natural for the study participant, however, the researcher must address a number of new safety concerns (Paterson, Gregory, & Thorne, 1999). Others must know your whereabouts, you must have access to emergency phone support, and you must have a clearly arranged "escape plan" if you find yourself in a situation in which your instincts tell you your safety may not be assured. While this might be self-evident to researchers entering studies of certain high-risk populations, it can be less evident when there is no such explicit focus.

However, it is important to remember that when you enter the home of someone else, you are no longer on your turf, and surprises can occur.

Honoring Confidentiality

All researchers understand and submit to explicit requirements about confidentiality in relation to the process and product of the research. Beyond those explicit requirements, however, there is a "gray zone" associated with the kind of information that may come your way when successfully working within a system. By its very nature, interpretive description uncovers perceptions rather than facts. In many instances, such as when studying persons with health conditions, you are likely to encounter perceptions and information about other patients, about individual clinicians, and about systems and settings themselves. While it can be awfully tempting to tell clinicians how many wonderful things you have heard about their care from your study participants, know that this kind of disclosure breaches confidentiality just as much as if you were reporting their poor performance. In either instance, your report violates the trust that the setting has placed in how you will use the information that you gain access to through your interactions with their staff or clients.

At the outset of a study, it can be difficult to appreciate just how complicated institutional confidentiality can be. Your ethical approval and the documentation of your plan in the research proposal may be public domain information and the agency may be pleased to openly acknowledge your involvement. However, if and when findings that might reflect badly on the institution arise, you may be in a very difficult position if you have made a commitment to disclose the name of the institution. For this reason, many researchers find value in using multiple settings, and in being oblique in their references to specific institutions (for example, calling it "a comprehensive tertiary-care center in a large Western Canadian province"). In a field such as health care, especially having entered your study on behalf of patients, it can be easy to find fault with systems like those involved with health-care delivery. However, do be aware that your "whistle blowing" may well jeopardize your study and those of subsequent researchers if you are not diplomatic, professional, and respectful in the manner in which you describe and interpret what you have seen and heard. It can help to remember that your ultimate goal is to engage systems in making constructive change, not alienating them from the findings you produce.

CHAPTER SEVEN

Constructing Data

The Process of Engaging with Data

Even as you begin the process of gaining entry into the field for your interpretive description study, you are already making that subtle shift between anticipating data collection and beginning to construct it. In the research proposal, you will have articulated clearly delineated processes of data collection and analysis, with specific steps and procedures for each, and then provided some explanation for the interrelatedness of those two steps within an inductively driven empirical inquiry. While you may have convinced your reviewers (and yourself) that you can keep these steps separate in your mind, you will find the actual practices of data collection and analysis much more complex than they might appear.

First, the idea that there are bits of data waiting out there to be harvested is something of a misnomer. The world is full of sights, sounds, smells, impressions, observations, and experiences, and you will be focusing your attention toward a particular species of these for the explicit purpose of obtaining knowledge about one particular phenomenon. Until you know that phenomenon quite well, you will not be able to accurately judge what is or is not a core ingredient of it and what might be influential upon it. You are therefore necessarily going to have to look broadly at the phenomenon, scanning a wide circle of possibly relevant information about it, as part of your process toward figuring out what you will consider it to contain, what will be related but more tangential, and what is only peripherally relevant. Thus, from the outset of your study, you are not "collecting" data as much as you are constructing an understanding of what constitutes data and how you will articulate it as such.

In the conventional descriptive research model, you would have carefully framed questions, and data would constitute whatever answers were provided to those questions (scores on scales, replies to interview questions, and so on). Those data collection techniques were designed at the outset to narrow the range of possibilities for what you were seeking and to minimize the researcher curiosity at probing further and exploring what might lie underneath the responses. In contrast, interpretive description explicitly capitalizes on the idea that surface answers are usually a bit misleading in the sense that they provide "top of mind" responses but not in-depth, rich, and nuanced understandings of what else is happening to explain those responses. Think of how normal discourse in society usually goes: In response to the question "Hi, how are you?" the typical rejoinder of "Fine" reveals absolutely nothing meaningful. So in interpretive description, we have the luxury of a method that allows us to dive into the muddy complexities that underlie those top of mind responses, to explore the contradictions and convolutions of human experience, and to render a kind of knowledge that informs us more deeply than is possible with a compilation of that which is easier to surface. While that too is important knowledge, it is not what drives us to interpretive description.

When we use the term "construction" in relation to the data collection process, we are explicitly drawing attention to the active role that the researcher is playing in deciding what of the universe of possibilities makes it into the data basket and becomes part of the later analytic considerations. However, by using that linguistic reference, we are also setting up something of a dilemma for the researcher, since the point of empirical research is not simply giving license to picking and choosing among available information to bolster a particular bias or preconceived opinion. We leave that for the journalist! Interpretive description provides us with a rationale for continually reflecting on the meaning of sitting in that middle philosophical position: I believe there may be something out there of common human subjective experience that can be known, and if I am to credibly uncover it, then the role that I will play in coming to know it is one for which I must be held highly accountable. It is this impeccable and meticulous accounting for one's intellectual processes through the data construction process that becomes the basis upon which "constructions" will eventually make the successful transformation from fabrications into meaningful "findings."

In this chapter, then, we'll explore in more detail the mechanics of data construction, and begin to consider some of the challenges that lie in store as you embark on your journey. Using some of the common data-collection techniques as a basis for reflecting on data construction in general, we'll focus on some of the pitfalls you might want to avoid and the motivations you'll want to maintain as the data construction process evolves. Because each study has its unique elements, and prescription is counterintuitive to an inductive reasoning process, what you'll find here is illustration of interpretive description logic in action within these various contexts. In each instance, the guidance you'll find will pertain to certain kinds of research questions, and it is always by returning to your own question that you'll be able to assure yourself that your own logical reasoning about process remains solid.

Options for Data Collection

Data collection in interpretive description can take many forms, and in fact the possibilities are infinite for creative researchers. Since subjective material tends to be fairly foundational to the kinds of questions that qualitative health researchers tend to ask, the goal in your data collection is figuring out an appropriate and defensible means by which to get as close to that subjective experience as you reasonably can so that you have a high probability of being able to access the kind of material that will allow you to answer your research question. The logic of deciding what your data source will be follows largely from a critical analysis of what's available to you, what the nature of that information will likely be (for example, its strengths and limitations), and how much credibility it offers as a reasonable foundation for any findings you might derive from it. So, for example, if you are considering using internet arthritis patient chat rooms as a source of data, you would be obliged to account for who it is they represent in this instance, and the basis upon which you understand them to reflect anything beyond the unique set of internet users who happen to have signed on to this specific site at that particular time. Under some circumstances, such sources could produce marvelous data, and under other circumstances they would be entirely meaningless. A solidly articulated logic, from the justification of your research question through to the design you set forth for answering it, will help ensure your eventual reader's assessment that your "findings" reflect knowledge and not nonsense.

All forms of qualitative data collection involve some particularities regarding what it is that they surface and what they might render invisible. Some are more obviously shaped by the researcher-subject interaction and context than are others, and some are more explicitly interpretive than others. It is imperative that you fully appreciate the implications of the data-collection strategy you are considering, and explicitly state its strengths and limitations from the outset. For example, if you are considering using art interpretation within your data collection approach, you'll want to ensure that you have a solid foundation not only in understanding what proponents of the method have written in its favor, but also what critiques have been leveled against it. Using an approach that inherently implies a highly subjective interpretation applied to the study of a highly subjective initial expression may offer you a distinct angle of vision on the phenomenon of interest, or it may lead you to findings that would speak more clearly to an art appreciation audience than they would to your intended audience of health care professionals, who we might say have no common *disciplinary* basis upon which to understand art interpretations as knowledge. Thus, rather than using art as your primary data collection mode, you might consider its utility as one complementary technique within your overall strategy to try to prompt different ways of revealing the kind of subjective material that is difficult to put into words.

Regardless of the data collection technique, it is essential that you inform yourself fully about its implications—not simply "the doing" but also the form of the data that may become available to you, the implications of analyzing and interpreting it, and the credibility that the data source will have for your eventual target audience. While using a wild and wonderful data collection strategy might sound like a lot of fun, you always need to keep your eye on your purpose for the study in the first place, and techniques that can be readily understood by members of the discipline are a reasonable place to start.

Interviewing

Much of what was addressed in the previous chapter pertains to the individual interview context and provides a basis upon which some of the challenges of interviews can be considered. Here, we'll address more explicitly the strengths and limitations of the interview as a primary data source, and some of the more common issues that arise in the conduct of data collection using interviewing.

Understanding Strengths and Weaknesses Interviews with individuals who have first-hand knowledge of a phenomenon have been the mainstay of qualitative health research for the past couple of decades. Because clinicians accept that there are aspects of any health or illness experience known only to the person going through it, they universally accept that "talking to the patient" is an essential element in pro-

---

TEXT BOX 7.1

Older Rural Women

Hayes used interpretive description methodology to generate an understanding of the vulnerabilities of older rural Appalachian women who lived alone and to better appreciate their need for formal and informal health support services. Documenting the accounts of these remarkable women as they shared their stories through interview, Hayes's findings depict a rural cultural tradition infused with a philosophy of life characterized by an intricate combination of self-reliance and community interdependence. Drawing on these women's homespun explanations and interpretations of their health management choices, Hayes provides us with a convincing appreciation for the central role that the meaning of "home" has in these women's lives and their preference for independently handling the natural health changes that occur with aging. These findings support the conclusion that, although formal social service and health resources may inadequately serve these women, they are deeply reluctant to accept assistance from the informal sources available within their families and communities. By understanding their approach to living, Hayes concludes that a better approach to conceptualizing systems of care can be created.

Hayes, P. A., (2006). Home is where their health is: Rethinking perspectives of informal and formal care by older rural Appalachian women who live alone. *Qualitative Health Research*, *16*(2), 282–297.

---

viding health care. Also, because time and focus to permit "in-depth" talking is rarely an option within a busy health care delivery system, the kinds of questions that qualitative health researchers often ask are those that might be answered if they had the luxury of more "talking time" with many of their patients in similar circumstances. Thus, the instinct for many researchers is that individual interviews will be their ideal data source.

Interviews are relatively easy to engineer and explain, and there is a wide body of available knowledge on how to conduct them effectively, both inside and outside of the qualitative research context (Fontana & Frey, 1994; Gilchrist & Williams, 1999; Hutchinson & Wilson, 1994; May, 1989; Miller & Crabtree, 1999b; Patton, 2002). Guidance on interviewing is usually relatively straightforward to obtain, since colleagues will have used the method, and the data collection technique feels familiar and comfortable to most health professionals and members of other applied disciplines. For these reasons, it has been argued that there is an overabundance of qualitative health knowledge derived from the individual "conversational" interview, and that a more informed analysis of the implications of that bias is needed (Nunkoosing, 2005; Silverman, 1998).

As pain researchers have long since discovered, it is difficult to fully reconcile the relationship between subjective and objective knowledge. In recognition that pain relief was not optimally provided on a widespread basis, some researchers have actively advocated for an entirely subjectively based reference point (such as the widely used definition, attributed to Margo McCaffery: "Pain is whatever the experiencing person says it is, existing whenever the experiencing person says it does") (McCaffery & Beebe, 1989, p.7). While we can all intuitively appreciate how useful this claim is in relation to our own pain, and would want our own health care providers to take our word for it rather than misinterpreting our stoic response to our discomfort, we also fully recognize that the subjective definition is highly vulnerable to manipulation if, for example, one wanted drugs for purposes other than normal pain relief. The pain example clearly illustrates the problem with the "either/or" position on subjective and objective knowledge in relation to these complex issues. And it is this complexity that underlies an important limitation to interviews that must be strongly acknowledged if an interpretive description is to remain true to its purpose.

Talking is one of our better and more accessible mechanisms for gaining access to that material we call subjective knowledge. At the same time, we all know that there are many human subjective experiences that are inarticulable, or that words cannot effectively convey. Further, we are well aware that "what" we talk about and "how" we talk about it are highly socially constructed. For example, while "the environment" has always existed, discourse about that environment required widely shared terminology referencing a conceptualization that was accessible to all. Even tiny children can now speak authoritatively about "the environment" where, for our great-grandparents' generation, putting forward ideas about the delicate relationship between humans and nature would have been fraught with much more challenge. In the modern sense, we are far more likely to reference conceptualizations that are familiar to us than to try to construct new ones. This means that those we interview are inclined to direct our attention toward what they think we will understand rather than that which most fully represents the complexity of their experience. Once talk show hosts glibly reference "family dysfunction" or "codependence," they become accepted conceptualizations with which individuals begin to make sense of and talk about the confusing set of thoughts and feelings they may long since have sensed but not expressed about their own web of interrelationships. What we can verbalize begins to shape what we are able to think about.

Because discourse is so intertwined with the dynamics of human social experience, it is quite easy for a qualitative health research interviewer to capture findings that, in effect, reflect simply the popular thinking of the times rather than something more deep, profound, and substantial about human experience. While documenting the kinds of temporal and contextual understandings that can be gleaned from discourse is quite useful (we might do well to be informed about how youth are linguistically referencing their alienation these days!), it is essential that we not confuse it with that other form of "subjective truth" that is thought to be independent of context and foundational to human experience. Qualitative researchers who rely heavily on interviews therefore must retain some humility about what it is they are uncovering, and have an obligation to reflect the particular relationship to time and place that their findings reflect. And this becomes one important reason for restraint in generalization, both in the doing of the research and in the reporting of the implications of your eventual findings.

Enhancing Quality If we engage in interviews with a strong consciousness of what has been told to us, on the basis of what conditions and prompts we have created for the interview, and with a thoughtful awareness of the broader social ideational context within which those interviews are conducted, we can certainly obtain a species of subjective knowledge that has relevance and importance for clinical application. In general, however, high-quality data will not simply be a product of posing questions and documenting responses. Rather, it will derive from a carefully thought out frame of reference, attitude, and communication style designed to build rapport (without stepping over the boundaries into friendship or therapy!), to elicit depth and clarification of threads within the account, and to foster elaboration, clarification, and even correction of your initial understandings and interpretations. It requires a substantial dose of humility and reflexivity to ensure that the dominant aspects of your own personality and passion don't steer the interactions in predictable directions. In essence, you are an encouraging and judgmentally neutral facilitator so that an individual can explain him or herself as fully as possible. Despite your years of clinical expertise and the months you may have spent reviewing the literature, you are entering the interview as a curious learner—confident that what really matters will be that which you are going to learn from the interview process. As your research progresses, you will find it natural and appropriate to effect more conceptual linkages between ideas within the accounts and the larger context of what you are learning. However, the core of what you are seeking is what can be expressed by the individual in his or her own context, way, and time.

Some practical matters associated with high-quality interviews are well worth mentioning. It goes without saying that you test your recording equipment in advance and are sufficiently comfortable with it to put your interviewee at ease. Especially when conducted in people's homes, interviews are prone to interruptions and unexpected shifts, so be prepared to accommodate those with grace and respectfulness. Most people simply must start their stories at the beginning, and you may well find that there is considerable introductory and background information that needs to be shared before your more focused inquiries become appropriate. Avoid impatience with this, as what you are hearing may turn out to have added value to you as you come to understand the phenomenon more deeply over time. Ensure that you have allowed sufficient time to be able to be present with the interview for the time that it takes to unfold. By all means take notes if you need to, such as jotting down key points to which you want to return, but ensure that your primary focus is on your participants, on listening and really hearing, on prompting further depth, on expressing your curiosity and genuine interest in the expertise that they are offering. When it comes time to end an interview, do provide something of a summary of key ideas in what you have heard, and share with that person what it is that you will be thinking about as you reflect further on what you've been told. If at all possible, build repeat interviews into your plan, so that your evolving interpretations can be informed by an increasing depth of clarifying questioning.

Interviews for the purpose of interpretive description will normally contain lots of contextual and background information of significance to your study participant that may not be entirely relevant to your intended purpose. The trick is to maintain a healthy respect for context, since you may not realize until much further along your analytic path that a particular contextual bit is in fact relevant in a way you might not have imagined. At the same time, it is also important not to confuse context with data. For example, in a study of breast cancer treatment experience, patients may universally feel compelled to begin their story with an account of their diagnostic experience. Recognize that this does not mean that the diagnosis overshadows the treatment experience, but rather that there may be a strongly shared sense of ensuring that you understand context.

As we discussed in Chapter 4, health professionals who interview regularly in the course of their practice often find it particularly difficult to shift into research-interview mode. They may find themselves feeling awkward and inhibited, and it may take time and practice to develop competence at qualitative research interviewing. Another common experience is to find that interviews fall dramatically short of the rich, articulate, and powerful stories that you had anticipated hearing. Not all people who have an experience will have the interest or inclination to wax poetical about it, and sometimes human expression can seem stuck in the mundane. Rather than showing your frustration with an interview participant because he or she is not giving you "good data," it is wise to keep focused on your curiosity about who this person is and why he or she is telling you what is being told. Sometimes the germs of an important new insight come from the voices that you would least expect.

Focus Groups

Focus groups should not be thought of as convenient ways to conduct individual interviews efficiently, but rather ways of capitalizing on group process to generate certain kinds of social knowledge, such as the beliefs and attitudes that underlie behavior (Brown, 1999; Carey, 1994; Krueger, 1988; Morgan, 1988; Stewart & Shamdasani, 1998). By understanding what they signify and what they are capable of yielding, you'll be able to judge when and how focus group data will enhance your inquiry as a primary or collateral method.

Understanding Strengths and Weaknesses With individual interviews, because you come away with a profound sense of unique and distinct stories, it can sometimes feel as if you are misrepresenting them when you try to summarize commonalities. With a focus group, you have the opportunity to meet distinct individuals each with some experiential knowledge about a phenomenon and see what happens when they engage in interaction with one another. Because the social dynamic of a focus group is the element that you are trying to generate, the method works best where your question is one with social dimensions to which each individual might contribute. For example, if you were curious about which model of support services might be best received by family caregivers of patients with a particular condition, you might structure a focus

TEXT BOX 7.2

Foreshadowing Aging

Using an interpretive description approach to guide data collection and using focus groups, Giddings and colleagues explored the experiences of "almost old" (i.e., 50–65 years) women with a range of chronic conditions. They were interested in understanding the changing context of the aging process among this group of women and documenting common pathways into the aging trajectory. What they found was that living with a chronic disease had prepared these women for the aging process. Their resourcefulness and expertise in coping with their conditions had produced a comfortable familiarity with how bodily changes influenced their ways of being in the world. For them, aging seemed a "matter of fact" phenomenon rather than a dreaded life event. Nevertheless, their anticipation of future bodily changes also made them aware of their vulnerabilities and conscious of the intricate balance of dependencies upon which their future wellbeing might rest. The authors felt that these insights would be valuable for health care professionals in building effective relationships that could support these women through the coming years.

Giddings, L.S., Roy, D.E, Predeger, E. (2007). Women's experiences of aging with a chronic condition. *Journal of Advanced Nursing, 58*(6), 557–565.

group that would capitalize on their analysis of the experience, observe a debate of the relative merits of the options, and ascertain whether your groups do or do not come to a comfortable consensus about preferences. The data you would be eliciting then is not so much a forced concession, but an understanding of whether or not opposite perspectives would be likely to disadvantage certain kinds of people depending on the model available. Thus, the focus group methodology allows you to go beyond "averaging" what individual contributions might suggest and exploiting the creative potential of interaction among perspectives.

A risk with focus groups is that in the wrong hands they can quite easily obscure nondominant perspectives and become something of a coercive data-collection mechanism. Because they are inherently social, they privilege the kinds of data that people tend to feel more comfortable expressing in the social domain, and substantial private, "politically incorrect," or diverse material would be unlikely to surface. Because few health professional researchers are posing questions for which the dominant public response is the only relevant one, focus group data must be considered with caution. In practice, many health professional researchers blend a design that solicits common aspects of a phenomenon but also explicitly solicits and acknowledges the validity of individual differences. Thus the focus group becomes one that informs the individuals within it about the others, and capitalizes on that broader base to try to generate group understandings that become the data.

Enhancing Quality   Focus groups work best if they are not large (six to eight individuals might normally be considered an upper limit) and if they are carefully orchestrated. Confidentiality and respectfulness must be assured, and the researcher/facilitator is obliged to maintain a strong control over what transpires in order to protect all members. Excellent broad-based and more targeted questions greatly enhance the capacity of the group to "focus," and a skilled group facilitator can create an environment in which group members genuinely address one another instead of sequentially speaking to the investigator. Effective leaders will also ensure a reasonable balance among participants in the competition for air time, drawing out those who are more reticent and skillfully guiding those who are more verbose. Because voices can be difficult to distinguish on audiorecording, many researchers choose to have an observer/note taker track the dialogue and identify who says what. Such field note support frees the facilitator to engage fully in steering the dialogue toward a productive conclusion.

If focus groups are to become a primary data source, careful reflection on their nature and constitution is especially *important* and a thorough accounting for these will become a major component of your credibility platform. In particular, it is essential to remain mindful of the manner in which the social dynamic of the group will have shaped the thinking of its individual members in various ways, and to ensure that the findings you come up with on the basis of your analysis remain true to that reactivity.

Participant Observation

In contrast to the interview, which seeks to gain close access to the language cues that help expose subjective experience, and the focus group, which seeks to exploit the social constructions within which we experience our subjectivities, observation provides a platform from which to reflect upon behavior and context (Bogdevic, 1999; Patton, 2002). As such, it too has dimensions that must be well understood for observation to become a credible source of interpretive description data (Adler & Adler, 1994; Mays & Pope, 1995; Mulhall, 2003).

TEXT BOX 7.3

The Context of Medical Dominance

Kenny and Duckett used interpretive description to better understand the context of medical practice in rural Australian hospitals during a time of significant policy revision. Interviewing key informant hospital administrators and clinicians from 20 rural hospitals, they were able to illuminate the manner in which medical relationships have been shaped by bureaucratic structures, medical shortages, medical entrepreneurs, and alternative service provision. In so doing, they depicted the consistent struggle that rural hospitals face to maintain adequate services and the challenging relationships that exist between rural hospitals and the physicians upon whom they are dependent. Their findings extend our understanding of how social interactions in a particular context can serve to perpetuate medical dominance and control as new models of care delivery emerge.

Kenny, A., & Duckett, S. (2004). A question of place: Medical power in rural Australia. *Social Science & Medicine, 58,* 1059–1073.

Understanding Strengths and Weaknesses Observation offers the distinct advantage of allowing you to sidestep the powerful effects of language and social influence. Just as none of us is capable of seeing ourselves exactly as we seem to others, direct subjective expression is well understood to obscure certain taken-for-granted elements of the meaningful world. Thus, being able to stand back from the self-consciousness with which individuals articulate their realities permits a researcher to pose a different set of questions pertaining to what people seem to be doing rather than what they say they think they are doing. As a strategy for gaining contextual understanding of the world within which subjective and social experience exist, observation can be a marvelous adjunct to your study or a data collection strategy all on its own.

A major weakness of observation is that you can't really know what aspects of the context are as taken for granted by you as they are for the actors within the setting. Thus, it can be challenging to sort out what it is that you are or are not observing and why. Unless you are concurrently obtaining other forms of data that would allow you to access perceptions, observation only reveals what is being done and not why it is being done in that manner. What conventional ethnographers understood about observation was that it was best accomplished with some clarity as to the levels of analysis that were being employed.

Thus the most comprehensive observational studies explicitly recognized both distinctions between and interrelationships among micro, meso, and macro levels of activity.

Enhancing Quality A well-known problem with observation is its reactivity, in that by observing something you bring it to the attention of those who exist within it in some manner that may not have been accessible before your arrival. Further, researchers unfortunately do sometimes forget that they are not the primary actors within the original setting and their own subjective experiences in the conduct of research are not equivalent to those of the primary actors. Thus, various forms of blurring of roles and positions is something that observers do need to attend to throughout their studies.

In order to conduct observation as effectively as possible, you'll need clear understandings as to the boundaries and scope of your study, and an ongoing process for feedback as to the effect you are having upon the setting. You may well find that periods of immersion and distance are essential both to maintain the equilibrium of the setting and to permit you to move between analytic levels. Meticulous documentation and recording are essential, and observational studies tend to rely heavily on reflective field notes to track the evolving logic that is shaping that which enters and exits your window of concern.

As is evident from these very brief comments, every data source and method of data collection has its advantages and drawbacks, and the researcher must be well aware of these in order to ensure that the logic of the research remains intact from the outset and through to the final conclusions. Recognizing this, many researchers consider triangulation of multiple data collection approaches to be a viable option within an interpretive description study. Adding an element of participant observation can help remind you that there may be multiple perspectives on an issue, rather than just the subjective one you are focusing on. Interviewing a few key informants for elements of meaning and context can help you reduce the possibility of misinterpreting what you see in your observations. And bringing together a focus group of individuals with whom you have had a series of individual interviews to stimulate their interpretation of commonalities and differences can powerfully refine your grasp of the phenomenon you are studying. In some instances, you will consider one source of data primary and the others more collateral, and in others you may design a study from the outset as explicitly capitalizing on the distinct angles of vision supported by different data collection strategies.

Regardless of your data collection method(s), your understanding of interpretive description will provide considerable guidance in how you work with and apply the principles that derive from the in-depth data collection resources to which you have access. Your applied orientation will help you retain a focus on what meaningfully becomes data and the complexities associated with decisions as to what you are looking for and how to find it. You understand that your position within the data field is one of description (with as much depth and richness as possible) and interpretation (in the sense of an ongoing reflection about what these data might mean). That methodological direction will also steer you away from predicting or projecting, from leaping to premature conclusions, or to "explaining" in the sense of generating theory. Rather, your understanding of the needs of the clinical world, as framed in your original research question, will help keep you on a decisional path that ensures the integrity of the data you construct and the credibility of the conclusions you make on the basis of it.

Managing the Collection

Regardless of your data collection approach, you will need an explicit plan for how you are going to manage data (Easton, McComish, & Greenberg, 2000). Data management has to do with tracking, organizing, and sorting what you bring from the field, and ensuring that it takes the form of material that you will be able to access and use throughout your data collection and analytic processes.

Protecting Data

Field notes and transcriptions of audio-recorded data tend to be the mainstay of interpretive description, although the principles of managing them would apply equally to collateral sources such as videotapes, photographs, or documents. First, you must scrupulously attend to the specific requirements of your ethics board with respect to such matters as identification and protection of confidentiality. Identifying information typically includes names and contact information, but may also in some studies include other material that could identify unique individuals, such as those that might have a rare disease or circumstance. Further, data tend to be messy in the sense of including lots of other potentially identifiable material (the name of the surgeon who did the procedure, the name of an institution where care was provided), and it is useful at the outset to clean these from notes and transcripts and replace them with more generic identifiers such as "surgeon" or "clinic". Original notes and tapes that do contain these identifiers should be carefully stored in a secure place, and separated from the sanitized copies that you will use for your own ongoing reference and analysis.

Beyond these fundamental protections, also ensure that any clerical support people who might have access to original material have committed to confidentiality (a signed agreement is advisable), and that mechanisms for sharing data among research team members or supervisors do not expose the data to going astray or being misused. Consider password-protected files and other means to ensure that access is tightly controlled and copies are not circulating out there in the internet ozone.

Sorting and Organizing

Qualitative data have a tendency to expand exponentially, and many researchers find themselves overwhelmed with volumes of information quite quickly. Thus, it is important to plan for how you will manage and organize data, how you will track your transcription, filing, and coding sequences, and how you will ensure both security and ease of retrieval. Some researchers feel a tendency to try to break down, summarize, and synthesize very quickly, and may need reminders to ensure that the contextual whole is preserved for ongoing analysis. If you too quickly extract only those key ingredients that you think will be relevant, you are likely thwarting your ability to move beyond where you first began. Other researchers will find just the opposite. By wanting to preserve and honor the integrity of the whole, they may find themselves incapable of sorting and organizing. It seems best to discover which kind of person you seem to be in this circumstance, and then create an explicit plan to overcome the potential limitations of your inclinations in this regard.

A marvelous adjunct to the data management process is the readily available assortment of qualitative research software. Such programs create various processes whereby data are entered into the software in a form that is highly amenable to organization and sorting, and, ideally, reorganization and resorting as your emerging analytic insights become apparent. Despite the enthusiastic claims of some of the manufacturers, however, you must always remember that such systems cannot conduct inductive analysis. What they are good for is putting data into groupings and structures that will remove some of the "grunt work" associated with conventional manual sorting and organizing;

providing you with access to that data in groupings and formats might facilitate your inductive analytic process. Because the volume of data is likely to be extensive and the meticulous attention required to code it notoriously exhausting, many newer researchers find it easy to get bogged down in the detail such that they cannot rise above it to actually analyze. So the main principle involved in working with any data-management system is that it be supportive of your analytic process, not a replacement for it. If it is so overly complex, time consuming, and structured that you can't step back and think about data, then it may be detrimental to your process. Until you are well familiar with the interaction between software programs and your own particular analytic and conceptual style, it is worth exercising some caution.

Although reliance on software is rapidly becoming the norm, do consider the possibilities inherent in basic word-processing programs, especially if you are a newer researcher conducting a smaller study. Just as different people are characteristically more linear or lateral in their thinking, researchers will find that they have certain kinds of analytic preferences when confronted with an evolving and growing body of fascinating material. Until you know your style, and can effectively match it with the capacities of a software-processing system, experimentation with paper and pencil, basic on-screen highlighting and filing techniques, or wall-chart graphics can help ensure that your inductive reasoning ability isn't overwhelmed by the directionality that each software program favors and you remain in control of your data construction and analysis.

Tracking Constructions

Although we will have the opportunity to engage more deeply in considerations of data analysis in the next chapter, the interpretive description method implies that you are engaging in it and data construction somewhat concurrently, and that analysis is what is informing your ongoing data construction. Because of this, an important element in managing your data is carefully documenting what has been gathered and thought about, and finding ways to track the evolution of each within your process over time. Some researchers refer to an "audit trail" as a feature of your eventual research report that will be requisite to the credibility of your findings. This means that you have provided your eventual audience with sufficient information about the decisional processes you made along the way to be able to recreate the logic whereby the data exist in the way that they do and the analytic process takes its eventual shape.

The hard work of data analysis relies on the intellectual practices associated with seeing possible relationships among pieces of data you are gathering and then considering the manner in which these relationships play out (or don't) across the growing and evolving wider data set. It isn't a passive activity, in that you are required to actively solicit further examples, variations, and contrasts in order to eventually conclude that patterns or themes exist and have relevance. However, when we are actively engaged in this kind of inductive reasoning process, we tend not to be overly disciplined about it. Most of us either leap to assumptions and become invested in them a bit too quickly or, conversely, become a bit paralyzed with the insecurity of articulating any linkage when we don't have a complete data set. The former will need to learn to slow up, document and reflect on their decisional points, and the latter will need to use their reflective documentation to create a safe space for trying out their conceptualizations. In either instance, careful journaling or note taking of some kind will be essential to being able to ask yourself later on "how is it that I came to that understanding?" and to produce a reasonable and defensible answer. This self-awareness of your evolving insights will eventually be reflected in the subtle language choices you make in writing up your findings and representing your conclusions. So an audit trail for your reasoning becomes an essential ingredient of the research enterprise.

By engaging with data, you enter into a discovery and creation process whose outcome remains somewhat tentative until you have almost arrived. You engineer a set of exposures whereby you have access to certain kinds of information about the phenomenon in which you are interested, and create a sequence of steps and activities that provoke your thinking mind to explore, question, seek, and tentatively interpret. Engaging with data in relation to a phenomenon about which you are concerned can be a powerful and thoroughly satisfying experience when well planned and executed. For many of us, it becomes a luxury not easily afforded to the world of clinical practice. And from this engagement, if you don't rush it too quickly and keep your eye on the eventual prize, you are creating the foundation for clinically meaningful new knowledge.

CHAPTER EIGHT

Making Sense of Data

The Work of Data Analysis

Generating new constructions out of the data you generate on the basis of your study is unquestionably the most painfully difficult and yet the most essential element in what constitutes a credible interpretive description study. Although it is relatively easy to enumerate what constitutes fundamentally flawed logic or entirely superficial analysis, the qualities that distinguish an elegant and convincing analysis from a mediocre one are much more difficult to pinpoint. While some of what might differentiate a brilliant from merely adequate analysis can be credited to the subjective response of the eventual audience, the expert researcher is one who knows how to make sense of data in a manner that does not simply defer credibility conclusions to the whim of the "theoretical reader," but rather explicitly engages that reader from the outset. By this I mean that the human mind, especially when stimulated by wonderful data, can make marvelous connections and associations. The scholarly mind knows how to distinguish between the various delightful experiential "ahas" that creative intellectual work produces so that he or she can generate products that reflect a strategic synthesis of new understanding. In other words, the reader is much less interested in how it is you came to an idea than what it is that you have to say. And when the researcher makes that message meaningful and relevant, it will be received as important insight.

This distinction between what the brain instinctively does with data and how data analysis ought to be conducted and reported is an important element in perfecting the art of data analysis in any qualitative research approach. Here we'll make reference to the kinds of "cookbook" data analysis approaches that are available in some of the qualitative research literature, examine something of how such techniques might inform our thinking or be useful in describing it to others, and reach beyond the stepwise guidelines into a consideration of some of the intricacies of thinking that can be tapped to develop the analytic muscle of which we humans are capable. Interpretive description requires an analytic form that extends beyond taking things apart and putting them back together again. It requires that we learn to see beyond the obvious, rigorously testing out that which we think we see, and taking some ownership over the potential meaning and impact of the visions that we eventually present as our findings.

In this chapter, then, we'll dive deeper into the hard work of data analysis, considering the core intellectual processes that you will use in engaging your mind to work with data and various practical techniques available to you for guiding the mysteries of analysis. We'll try to move you beyond formulaic approaches and toward fully exercising your innate analytic and conceptual capacities in turning data into credible and meaningful findings. By temporarily breaking down that process into component parts, we'll create a structure from which you can select approaches that are consistent with your unique disciplinary goals, the topic at hand, and your own particular analytic proclivities. We'll orient you to the location of the typical landmines that might derail your analysis or detract from its quality, and steer you toward the kinds of intellectual processes that are most likely to produce a successful interpretive description outcome—a meaningful, rigorous, and satisfying set of findings.

From Pieces to Patterns

Entering data collection, we tend to be bombarded with billions of possible bits of information that vie for our attention. It is important to remember that, as open-minded as we believe ourselves to be, we are already hardwired for highly selective organizing and sorting into what counts as meaningful. When the person we are interviewing references "anger," we immediately associate that with a conceptual category of "emotions" and assign it a negative valence. Often, we go much further and create value judgments around it, such as deciding whether it seems "justifiable" and "constructive" or not. Our antennae almost instinctively become attuned to detect other emotion signals, such that we notice, sort, and organize them more quickly when we have an emerging pattern for them to fit into. In most instances, the frame and tone of our ongoing interview style are shaped by what our antennae are expecting to detect and the emerging patterns that are forming in our subconscious thought.

The basis upon which each of us conducts this rapid-fire processing and sorting is a combination of our personality and experience, including our disciplinary orientation as well as our particular biases and curiosities. While we have many mechanisms by which to try to understand the former, the latter often take the form of mythical "trickster ravens" defying our conscious control. The process of developing experience and expertise as a qualitative data analyst is therefore very much one of learning technique and developing genuine insight, enjoying those tricksters but keeping them safely in their cages. We need a lot of knowledge of who we are in order to maintain some oversight of what we see within the data and consequently what sense we begin to make of it.

The initial phases of data analysis are very much a time of allowing ourselves to react to the initial pieces of data that seem to take on a life of their own and "attract" our attention. Within the thousands of words exchanged in the course of an interview, some choice words or phrases are very likely to "stick" in our minds—to take prominence in our attention and demand consideration. It is useful to reflect on why this occurs. First, our minds are necessarily primed with expectations of what we are likely to find when we make an observation or conduct an interview. That which is most likely to be memorable is either the prototypical case that fits the expectations or its diametric opposite. The mind is highly reactive to the unexpected, and we may well find that the "contrasting case" evokes the strongest sense of curiosity and delight, leading us to explore it in more depth and detail, and to find ourselves theorizing about why it has occurred. We then become sensitized to patterns that fit both the prototypical and the contrasting case, simply because we are now looking for them and have stimulated our sensitivities to notice them. Conversely, it is also possible for us to ignore or "block out" contrasting cases, simply because we don't hear or see them. Because we are already so focused in our attention, even when we intend to come into the field fully "open," our minds want to selectively disregard that which they feel is not among the stimuli that they are seeking to find. So an early aspect of the data analysis process involves making accurate records and spending time to be immersed in those records, developing a sense of the whole beyond the immediate impression of what it is that they contain.

Although it has become common nowadays to employ professional transcriptionists, I think that something has been lost in giving away that opportunity to really slow our attention to the nuances, words, phrases, and pauses, and to hear more deeply what the language contains. Thus, for neophyte researchers engaging in smaller studies, I often encourage some engagement in the transcription process as a means to enforce that shifting pace of attention that characterizes so much of our scholarly reading and reflection. It can be amazing what you hear when you focus on words and sounds and silent spaces rather than simply on storyline.

The Tradition of Coding From the earliest engagement in data collection, many authorities focus their analytic guidance on processes relating to coding the pieces of data so that they will later on be amenable to sorting into patterns, testing those patterns for relationships, and conceptualizing those relationships into findings (Crabtree & Miller, 1999b; Priest, Roberts, & Woods, 2002). This idea of attaching a "code" to a piece of interview transcript or field note derives from assumptions that one knows what the element entails, what other kinds of things might be similar, and what it ought to be distinguished from. Essentially, coding represents the initial basket into which the laundry is being sorted—dark versus light, and various shades of color, for example. However, as anyone who has experienced bringing two distinct laundry styles into an intimate relationship will have learned, there is a great deal more to the subjective judgment than simply detecting color shades. Different people's strongly held opinions about laundry will involve distinguishing natural fabrics from synthetics, color-fast from those requiring individual attention, and even items of washable clothing from those that ought not to have been placed in the laundry basket to begin with. In the case of laundry, the preliminary sort that may have been performed by one member is easily reversed when the family's chief laundry authority surveys the entire basket. However, once that initial load of laundry has begun in the wash, you become somewhat more limited in your options. In the case of data analysis, if an initial sort is based on entirely the wrong set of codes, the collection can quickly become sufficiently vast that it becomes impossible to undo the damage and beginning again at the beginning tends to be highly discouraging. This explains an element of the caution that was suggested against over-enthusiasm for data management software in the previous chapter. Like all good electronic games, these programs have compelling features, and you want to ensure that those features do not overshadow your use of reason, intelligence, and inductive thinking in driving the analysis. Premature coding and sorting are serious threats to analysis when researchers abdicate their full responsibility.

Caution aside, it is almost inevitable that some coding will be needed in order to sort and organize information into a manageable form. It can be instructive to consider some of the formal coding devices that have been generated in relation to other forms of qualitative research, and in some instances to draw inspiration (if not direct authority) from them. In particular, the most advanced coding guidance derives from the methodological tradition of grounded theory, within which three distinct forms of coding are widely applied (Glaser & Strauss, 1967; Strauss, 1987; Strauss & Corbin, 1998). Open coding involves "fracturing" the data—taking it apart and examining those discrete parts for the similarities and differences they reveal. This process helps to distinguish basic conceptual units within the data, delineate the properties that characterize them, and organize them into categories. Axial coding begins with the categorized conceptual data and creates the mechanism through which interactions among them can be worked out by identifying such properties as the conditions that give rise to them and the contexts within which they are typically embedded. It requires a formal testing procedure as these relationships are considered, drawing on existing data and ongoing data collection to verify the extent to which proposed connections hold true. Finally, selective coding occurs when axial coding has illuminated core categories to which all other subcategories relate and builds a conceptual framework from which to generate the new grounded theory. What becomes apparent when we consider the three forms of coding together is that they explicitly link the early analytic processes to the larger social purpose of the enterprise—building a coherent theoretical position that explains variation within the phenomenon (Strauss, 1995). This complex set of intellectual operations explains why grounded theory done properly is a massive proposition, and why selectively adopting a minor subset of the coding operations may not represent a satisfying analytic approach (Stern, 1994).

A good coding scheme is one that steers you toward gathering together data bits with similar properties and considering them in contrast to other groupings that have different properties. In interpretive description, because the objective is rarely at the fine-tuned level of words and expressions but far more often in the realm of themes and ideas, it is quite important not to be derailed by excessive precision in your early coding. For example, while you might initially notice expressions within the description of an illness experience that contain the word "depressed," your initial coding is likely to need to be sufficiently broad to also include "discouraged," "down," "sad," or even "not all that happy" in order that you can begin to grasp what the underlying shared intent might be within that collection of accounts. With a broad-based code, you will create a collection from which you can then begin to consider whether some of these refer to the illness itself while

---

TEXT BOX 8.1

Talking About Cancer

Lundgren and colleagues used a complex thematic analytic approach informed by interpretive description to explore intricate patterns in understanding of cancer revealed in interviews with women attending cervical screening clinics and the midwives who performed their pap smears as part of a national cancer screening initiative. They found that, although the midwives felt they had significant gaps in their cancer knowledge, they recognized that their role involved educating and informing patients about it. The research team observed that, while the women attending the cervical screening clinic often used the term "cancer" spontaneously in their interviews, the midwives tended to avoid it, preferring indirect references such as "changes in cells." The findings revealed that these midwives relied heavily on personal knowledge of cancer-related issues because they lacked professional guidance for this particular role. The authors concluded that the midwives' characteristic focus on wellness rather than pathology may make the routine cancer screening role a more difficult adaptation than it would be for nurses. The authors framed some recommendations for monitoring this aspect of the national screening program to ensure that it met its objective.

Lundgren, E.-L., Tishelman, C., Widmark, C., Forss, A., Sachs, L., Törnberg, S. (2000). Midwives' descriptions of their familiarity with cancer: A qualitative study of midwives working with population-based cervical cancer screening in urban Sweden. *Cancer Nursing*, *23*(5), 392–400.

---

others reference life events consequential to the illness, whether they reflect initial conditions or the trajectory of disease, or whether they reveal the profound emotion that is the central theme or contextual background to what seems to be the real story. Thus, in this example, the initial code is creating a mechanism by which you can bring together a group of data bits that *might* be thematically related (or might not) so that you can interrogate that collection, as well as the evolving data construction process, as to what those relationships might look like.

Taking this coding example further, by noticing early on in your study that many interview accounts did include such "meaning units," you might assign a "depressed" code to the collection, evolve your preliminary definition of the code to allow for a fairly wide inclusion, but still permit distinction from other kinds of data, and then keep the idea of "depressed" in play until such time as it seemed clear to you that the important underlying idea will be more meaningfully represented by quite different groupings and descriptors. If, by this time, you have invested a significant amount of time and energy carefully labeling all of the items within the "depressed" basket with their various terms and valences, you are naturally inclined to resist completely eliminating this code, and your mind is likely to want to bargain with you for retaining it and simply adjusting the term with which you reference it. This kind of compromise is precisely the pitfall against which I am advocating in encouraging you to use only the most broad-based and "generic" coding schemes until you have moved quite a distance down the analytic path and can more clearly see the implications of your increasingly explicit and fine-tuned coding sensibilities (Thorne, Reimer Kirkham & O'Flynn-Magee, 2004).

Unlike the fixed-form coding that is employed within deductive research traditions, coding within inductive research becomes an active process that allows you to experiment with trying different angles of vision from which to gaze upon the whole complicated collection of data bits so that you can begin to appreciate the implications of each of the available options for handling, grouping, and reconstructing pattern within them. Where coding fails to serve this purpose, and especially where it becomes a slave driver all on its own, it becomes fundamentally counterproductive to the process of generating good research findings. Research reports generated on the basis of premature coding tend to be "bloodless findings," in the sense that they offer nothing new or different from what we would have initially observed, and miss the opportunity to use structure as a means to elaborate meaning. Thus, coding is a tool to be used cautiously, critically evaluated at every stage of the analysis, and kept firmly in its place as a crude replica of the marvelous innate capacity we humans have to find the meaning that lies hidden within apparent chaos.

Alternatives to Coding Immersion in transcripts and field notes is often enhanced by the act of jotting down marginal memos or highlighting with colors to reflect apparent thematic similarities, and these devices are generally more consistent with the evolving analytic thought of interpretive description than are the more formal coding systems. "Coding" implies a certain term or signifier being applied or not applied to each data instance. It becomes strategic once you are highly confident that you do want to harvest all instances of a particular thing, and you can distinguish what does and does not fit the category. Long in advance of that certainty, however, you are going to want to "flag" for yourself certain data elements as potentially meaningful for various reasons. They might represent a model case of something you think may be important in your final conceptualization, a contrary case that seems different from all the rest, a particularly poignant or representative sample of something, or an element you have not previously encountered in other cases and want to ensure that you don't overlook. In many instances, simple "attention grabbers" are sufficient to ensure that these data bits aren't lost—you might use asterisks in your text margins or electronic flags in your files to ensure that your attention will be drawn to them on your next scan of the data, or you might want to cut and paste copies of them into a separate file housing a wide variety of bits that seem somehow important, later returning to ask yourself more informed questions about what they might mean in the context of your evolving inquiry.

Rather than thinking about your organizing structures as codes, which can reify them into a rigid structure before you realize it, you might consider using various kinds of group signifiers and language referencing devices to ensure that you are able to consider like elements together and begin to compare them with similar or unlike elements in the early phases of your data analysis. Sometimes explicitly assigning meaningless labels, such as "Category A Data," is helpful in that it explicitly defers inscribing meaning onto the grouping until you have moved further along your analytic journey. Similarly, strategies of bringing together potentially similar ideas in a mechanism that doesn't reflect a significant investment in formal coding can create subsets of the total data that allow you to reread, reflect, and hypothesize long in advance of determining what they are or how they will align within the final analysis. Word processing systems are especially useful for this purpose, allowing you to cut and paste into electronic files with descriptive titles that capture the nature of the collection without prematurely implying meaning. When using such systems, it is always wise to embed a location code (participant number, transcript page number) with perhaps further descriptive information (48-year-old married man with lung disease) so that you can quickly envision the larger context in which the initial data bit was contained and aren't tempted to consider it out of that context.

A factor that often steers us toward premature coding in qualitative research is the understandable urge not to lose those marvelous "quotable quotes" that we encounter within our data even before we necessarily know what meaning they actually illuminate. Often we hear an especially poignant account and "know" that it contains the seeds of an important insight that we feel compelled to ensure will be included in the final rendering. My recommendation is to flag and harvest those especially powerful pieces early in the data analysis process, perhaps creating a "quotable quotes" file. This strategy reassures us that they will not be lost and reduces the risk that their urgent claim upon our attention will overly dominate our evolving analytic structure. Being human (and qualitatively oriented), we are all suckers for the vivid anecdote; we know how powerfully they can communicate our message, and we also know how carefully we must handle them if they are to advance, rather than detract from, our scientific credibility. So give them their due from the outset, promise yourself they will find their way into the final report regardless of structure, and you will find that their individual voices become far less insistent within the chorus of analytic possibilities.

From Patterns to Relationships

Beyond organizing the data bits into various groupings, the work of analysis involves making sense of what relationships the various groupings have one to another, and inductively building some sort of coherent whole out of an iterative reasoning process as to the implications of understanding them in various ways (Miles & Huberman, 1994). If we get stuck on pattern or over-invested in a particularly elegant coding scheme, we are unlikely to fully exploit our intellectual capacity to consider relationships that break down our initial grouping structure. For example, if we have a wonderful collection of data bits that look like "coping strategy," we may find it difficult to step back and give up that grouping within our eventual organizational scheme, or to consider that grouping them in that manner may have misrepresented the overall experiential whole we hope to depict within our phenomenon. As soon as we have conceptualized coping strategy, we imply that there is a shared something to be coped with, that there is something volitional to responding to it, and that there are other responses that imply "not coping." We therefore may miss the opportunity to recognize that thinking about coping strategies may be our discipline's shorthand device for distilling from complex life experience that which we feel capable of influencing. And in so doing, we may recreate as findings our initial disciplinary assumptions that people need our help in particular ways.

Knowing Your Data To ensure that you move beyond the self-evident and superficial in linking the groupings and patterns within your data, you must consciously engage in various operations designed to shift your attention sequentially from individual cases to the whole data set, from groups of similarity within certain cases to various manifestations of difference within other cases. In so doing, you gradually begin to achieve increasing levels of clarity in your understanding of what relationships exist among instances within your data. In some instances, data elements that initially seemed disparate will become linked as you come to better appreciate the implications of their contextual meaning. In other instances, you will deconstruct the initial groupings you generated in favor of better and more comprehensive understandings. When I interviewed families with cancer, home visit interviews typically began with such requests as taking a tour of the garden, inspecting some antique furniture carved by a distant relative, or looking through an album of holiday photos. When my analysis evolved to the point where I understood these as powerful positioning statements on the part of these families (as in, "you can't possibly understand what cancer has done to us until you have a sense of who we are as a family"), then I became far better able to appreciate their role in our interviews and reflect their relevance throughout the ongoing interview process with these families. Rather than feeling impatient about yet another hundred photographs to review (and wanting to get on with "real" data collection), I was able to deepen my interviewing and concurrent analytic process with the insight that all aspects of the cancer experience were informed by the self-defined understanding of family life that each was so intent on preserving in spite of cancer.

As with the general sorting and organizing of data into patterns, the process of extending pattern recognition into an understanding of relationships requires active and thoughtful engagement in the work of analysis. Once you understand what it is that you are trying to achieve at each level of the analysis, you are better armed to appreciate the significance of various strategies and techniques that may be recommended in the literature. Generating a range of operations to enact upon your interesting bits of data is likely to be an evolving process until such time as you have familiarized yourself with your own mental proclivity and your visual/spatial preferences for data display. The technique used by your dissertation supervisor may not work at all well for you, and rigid adherence to the formal guidelines offered within the qualitative data-analysis literature may feel hollow and ritualized rather than creative and inspirational. What you are aiming for is a series of technical and/or intellectual operations that will allow you to know your data intimately, to consider similarities and differences with respect to a wide range of dimensions among the various cases you have included in your sample, and to follow a logical line of inquiry in relation to individual cases as they illuminate those aspects that might legitimately be considered patterns and themes within the data set overall.

TEXT BOX 8.2

The Challenge of Hormone Replacement Therapy

Reece used interpretive description to better understand why many women discontinue their prescribed hormone replacement therapy despite awareness of established evidence of its health benefits. Analyzing interview data from women who had made various choices in this regard, Reece learned that the experiences of women on HRT commonly included the impact of both physical and emotional effects of the hormones, concerns about those effects, and not being heard when they expressed their concerns to professional health care providers. Those who discontinued hormone therapy attributed that decision to a wide range of somatic and psychological experiences combined with an informed critical analysis of the evidence associated with its relative value in comparison to the hassles associated with continuance. In most respects, Reece found that the perceptions of women who remained on the hormones and those who had discontinued were quite similar, and it was the unpleasantness of the side effects that tended to tip the balance. On the basis of these findings, Reece was able to identify a variety of ways in which the insensitivity of the health care system seemed to contribute to their dissatisfaction and discontinuation of the therapy.

Reece, S. M. (2002). Weighing the cons and pros: Women's reasons for discontinuing hormone replacement therapy. *Health Care for Women International, 23,* 19–32

Borrowing Technique The available body of literature on various qualitative approaches provides some valuable stepwise options to working with data so that patterns and relationships become observable. Grounded theory has contributed "constant comparative analysis," an approach whereby you compare every piece of data (an interview, a statement, a theme) with all others that may be similar or different from it in order to theorize all possible relations among data (Glaser & Strauss, 1967). Such analytic approaches are best suited to studies in which the purpose is to uncover commonalities and patterns across cases within human experience (Thorne, 2000a). Within this grounded theory tradition, there are examples of highly prescriptive techniques for conducting constant comparative analysis (e.g., Strauss & Corbin, 1998). While such recipes may prove comforting to new researchers in that they create the illusion of a manageable sequence of operations, uncritical reliance on them tends not to be consistent with the highest levels of analysis.

Phenomenology offers a rather different analytic strategy, since its purpose is to discover the underlying structure or essence of a phenomenon (Colaizzi, 1978; Giorgi, 1985; Ray, 1994; Van Kaam, 1969). This approach typically challenges the researcher to set aside preconceptions so that entirely new conceptualizations can be inductively derived from the deep study of specific cases. Although they vary in the extent to which interpretation is an acceptable element, all of the phenomenological approaches strive for a rich description that illuminates deep essential structure of human experience.

Ethnographic methods tend to provide a systematized set of patterns within which new data are analyzed and interpreted. These patterns derive from the fundamental assumptions held by anthropology and sociology about human social organization (belief systems, kinship patterns, ways of distributing resources, and so on) (Gubrium, 1988). The analytic process, then, becomes one of sorting observations into these predetermined general categories, searching for inconsistencies and contradictions and generating increasingly integrated conclusions about what is happening and why.

Narrative and discourse analysis also invoke distinct data-analysis processes. While both draw our attention to linguistic representations of human experience, they rely on different aspects of that representation as a source of meaning. Narrative approaches tap the order and organization we humans give to cognitively unstructured life experiences when we articulate them in a communicable form (Muller, 1999; Sandelowski, 1994b). Discourse analysis recognizes speech as an explicit linguistic tool that has been devised on the basis of various social influences, and orients us toward understanding what else is represented in the various ways in which people communicate ideas (Boutain, 1999).

Beyond these explicit qualitative methodological traditions, one can also draw analytic inspiration from many other specific interpretive techniques that have been generated to address particular kinds of questions. As Feldman (1995) explains, ethnomethodologists seek out processes by which people make sense of the institutions through which they live and the interactions they have within them; semioticians seek surface manifestations and the underlying structures from which they denote meaning; and deconstructionists look for the multiple meanings that are implicit within events, conversations, or texts. In relation to each of these explicit purposes, interesting analytic maneuvers have been articulated that may be applicable for researchers using interpretive description to study specialized topics.

Within the literature of each of these methodological and analytic traditions, the reader can find excellent examples of analytic guidance that enhance analysis in the interpretive description context. Indeed, a robust, mature program of interpretive description research may ultimately draw inspiration from techniques devised from a wide range of these approaches. What distinguishes interpretive description, however, is that none of these approaches is borrowed uncritically or used in a manner that is entirely faithful to the original tradition. Instead, the researcher using an interpretive description approach remains mindful of his or her obligation to account for the relationship between the technique and the underlying approach to what constitutes knowledge from which it has been extracted. This ensures that attention to technique does not degrade the analytic process into a collection of empty categories that will have limited usefulness for the generation of new knowledge (Silverman, 1993).

Documenting Analytic Thinking Beyond using visual and syntactic reference points as a means of becoming familiar with what your data set contains, I recommend that you create a set of analytic notes that will allow you to ask increasingly complex questions about what it all might mean. Although analytic memos can take many forms, I personally prefer a blank notebook into which you can enter dated collections of thematic lists, pose questions among cases, and jot down emerging patterns that you wish to track. The advantage of the blank page is that it invites you to engage with it in a new format each time you write. Today's entries might look like "ways of . . ." or "kinds of . . ." descriptions, while tomorrow's might look like trigger questions for your ongoing analytic reasoning such as "I wonder if . . .?" or "Have I seen other cases of . . .?" Some of us think in taxonomies of word lists, others in visual "bubbles and arrows," and the blank notebook permits experimentation with a range of representations that can make manifest your evolving thought and inquiry. During regular brainstorming periods, it is wise to jot down every key element that you think you may be seeing. Reviewing what you have written and allowing your interpretive mind to ask questions of it repeatedly, you can engage your thinking toward grouping, connecting or highlighting these more disjointed early entries. From what begins as random bits, you are gradually able to see the beginnings of order and organization take shape over time, not through some magical process but with the benefit of your disciplined critical reflection and continual interpretive challenge. When you have documented the complex stages through which your thinking evolves as you come closer to fully formulated analytic conclusions, you begin to feel a real sense of ownership over the eventual structure that your findings will take, and your research becomes a convincing product of that process.

Over time, the use of such an intensive analytic memo process tends to increasingly refine a set of ideas that play a progressively more important role in your ongoing data collection process, sensitizing you to explore further for expansion and clarification when one of these ideas is casually referenced in conversation, and to seek contrary or different cases as you encounter more instances within the real world. While you may find that you begin with dramatically different ideas as to what might constitute an important observation or an emerging relationship between data pieces, over time you are very likely to find that certain ways of thinking about these become more compelling and reflective of those elements you are discovering that simply must be told. Becoming truly committed to the eventual analytic structure that will best serve your findings requires that you fully appreciate its implications and enable you to clearly identify its advantages over other organizational structures you might have considered to showcase the various data elements. So throughout the organizing, conceptualizing, writing up, and presenting phases, you'll appreciate that you committed this internal dialogue onto paper rather than trying to reconstruct it from memory.

Data Analysis in Play

Although data analysis is justifiably depicted as excruciatingly hard work, it is important not to get so caught up in the tough slogging that you forget to enjoy the marvelous intellectual adventure you are on. For the researcher who has taken up interpretive description in order to address a clinical problem and learn more about a phenomenon central to professional practice, it is imperative, after you have spent (most likely) months reviewing the literature, developing your research proposal, entering the field and gathering data, not to lose sight of the passion and curiosity that brought you into the inquiry in the first place. The enormity of the effort it takes to bring you to the data analysis stage is part of what makes data analysis so difficult, and it is important to ensure that you avoid feeling overwhelmed with exhaustion and overeager to finish up your research project quickly. The difference between an excellent research product and one that is mediocre or worse depends on your capacity to reignite the flame of enthusiasm and fully engage in making sense of the hard-earned data you have before you. For this reason, it is essential to plan on a signifi-cant investment of time in the data analysis phase, and to ensure that you find ways to charge up your batteries to sustain your energy for the duration.

In the above discussion of the "work" of data analysis, I made a fairly strong argument against early or excessive coding because of the effects it can have upon the capacity to see beyond the codes and the enthusiasm you can muster for considering alternative angles of vision that might better illuminate the analytic problems you are thinking about. My motivation was to help you avoid the burden of having in-vested so much time in coding that you become unwilling to abandon your initial system, and also to keep your attention on the inductive analytic capacity of your mind as the primary source of fuel for the analytic process. Despite the rhetoric that you might read in some re-search reports, findings never "emerge" from the data on their own, and if they are to be worth something in the end, they always come about because a human mind has engaged strategically and construc-tively in the business of active analysis. One way of ensuring that you rise above the drudgery and keep your mind lively and in control is to find ways to take delight in the process, to trigger your innate curiosity, and to follow the many lines of fascinating inquiry that your induc-tive processes illuminate. What you are trying to achieve is what May (1994) refers to as an acquired aptitude for "magic." Here we'll consider two ways of keeping your mind lively through the analytic process—using various techniques to avoid the tricky hazards along the pathway, and sustaining momentum toward the goal.

Avoiding Hazards

As is the case with all qualitative methods, data analysis in interpre-tive description is full of potential traps into which the inexperienced and unsuspecting researcher is prone to falling. As has often been ob-served (Morse, 1994b; Priest et al., 2002; Wolcott, 1994), it is typically much easier to explain what not to do than to fully articulate what to do—at least in a manner that is foolproof! Most experienced qualitative researchers have developed their interpretive instincts on the basis of errors—sometimes hard-earned insights obtained at considerable cost. Paying attention to the patterns of these errors, and using that aware-ness to heighten your reflection at decision points along the analytic path can help keep you from having to learn them all on your own, and at the potential expense of research quality. Here we review some of the main landmines in inductive analysis (Thorne & Darbyshire, 2005) so that, with any luck, you can strategically avoid stepping on them and reach your destination safely.

Premature Closure Perhaps because the specter of analysis creates such anxieties in the minds of neophyte researchers, a primary threat to meaningful findings becomes stopping at the first major *"aha!"* Once that kind of major experiential insight occurs within an analytic process, it can be tempting to assume that this is all there is, and that it is both meaningful and important. Using this first flash of understanding as the basis for all further interpretation can produce premature closure on what might be there in the data and prevent you from fully exploiting what you have available to develop the most intricate and conceptually linked interpretations possible.

A second route toward premature closure on what you see in your data comes from what can be termed "overdetermination of pattern." This can occur when the researcher's mind creates artificial coherence among data pieces and patterns, often basing those linkages on relatively superficial elements within the phenomenon. If the data seem to "fit" overly quickly, it is most likely that the issues around which they fit will be those that have been primed in your thinking by the literature or experiential knowledge you brought into the study in the first place (Kearney, 2001).

Misinterpreting Frequency Another kind of interpretive error is the assumption that, if things occur frequently within a data set, they are necessarily more relevant or important. In much of human discourse, we frame our meaningful communications within the context of socially constructed frameworks and rule sets, and being able to distinguish the medium from the message is an essential element of transforming data into findings. Picking up on an earlier example, if, in response to the greeting "Hi, how are you? " most of your study participants respond with "Fine, thank you," the uniformity of that response tells you considerably more about social expectations than about their actual state of health.

The opposite kind of interpretive error is that, having encountered one particularly graphic instance of a thing, you assume it probably happens often, even though you haven't actually seen any other cases within your sample. This "trick of the mind" may reflect an unconscious attempt to ensure that your findings extend beyond what has previously been reported and are truly original and novel. While a surprising bit of data is well worth careful attention, and working at it analytically may lead you toward new ways of thinking about relationships within the data, it is always important to interrogate yourself honestly with regard to what you would need to do, see, or learn in order to be able to extend the observation into something worthy of the status of "finding."

Yet another variation of the frequency problem is the assumption that, because you haven't seen something, it doesn't exist. As you exploit data for patterns and relationships, you begin to become painfully aware that your data set likely does not include all of the possible variations that you hoped it might, and that the better you understand the data, the more complex the problem of variation becomes.

Over-Inscription of Self As was discussed in Chapter 3, a number of analytic problems can occur if you aren't careful about the extent to which you, the researcher, have "become one with" the data. While your engagement with study participants has undoubtedly created the context within which excellent data could emerge, the extent to which this represents skilled interviewing, the study participants' relief at being heard, or some other dimension of your interaction with them can be difficult to sort out. Because you may be learning intimate details about amazing lives, it is tempting to think that you have been entrusted with data that are especially rich by virtue of the special relationships you have formed with your study participants and, as a consequence, you have become an important part of the story.

Although human interaction characterizes the environment in which data are obtained, apparent self-absorption (or what Sandelowski and Barroso (2002) have termed "hyper-reflexivity") will detract dramatically from the credibility and impact of your findings. It is therefore a good idea to poke a little fun at yourself if you find you are starting to take yourself too seriously, and to find safe and friendly self-reflective strategies for keeping yourself out of the way of your research.

Each of these hazards can lead to a misrepresentation of meaning that can seriously complicate your capacity to arrive at credible and meaningful findings. When you get to the analysis stage, therefore, it becomes especially important to afford yourself the time to step back from time to time, create some distance from the process, and take advantage of every opportunity to challenge the intellectual linkages you find yourself beginning to formulate. You might find it useful to read about the typical analytic traps into which researchers fall (Baker, 2006; Miller & Crabtree, 1999c; Silverman, 1993; Thorne & Darbyshire, 2005) or compare notes with others who have experiential knowledge of the analytic process. What you are trying to do is keep yourself honest and keep the analytic momentum moving forward.

Approaching the Goal

Although it is incredibly important to attend to avoidable hazards that might derail you from your larger purpose, it is equally important not to be immobilized by the enormity of the task and the complexities of the challenge. In these concluding remarks about the data analysis process, we'll focus on some techniques and strategies to keep yourself moving systematically toward the goal of a coherent, defensible, and data-grounded descriptive interpretation of the phenomenon you have set out to study.

The overarching intellectual task driving your data analysis journey in an interpretive description study is making sense of which ideas are core to the phenomenon you are studying and which are more usefully understood as context. That is, you are trying to sort through which ideas are fundamental to an understanding of the phenomenon about which you have posed your question, and which may be common, and even important, but are essentially part of some other story or question. In other words, you are seeking a way to rationalize the boundary between these two options.

Confirming your Bases   As your mind moves from data to pattern and from pattern to relationship, you need to continually find ways to confirm or challenge the basis upon which your mind is making linkages between the pieces and parts within the data. Stepping away from the data to ask yourself "What am I seeing?" and "Why am I seeing that?" forces you to acknowledge that there is much else to be seen and that alternative lenses might have generated slightly or even substantially different perspectives on what was there to be found. What you will typically recognize is that, in the midst of an effective data analysis process, you will cycle between periods of supreme confidence in what you are interpreting and other periods of profound doubt that you can find anything meaningful within the overall chaos. Don't despair, because this subjective experience of data analysis is a positive sign that your critical mind hasn't failed you, and a helpful reminder that interpretive description findings don't come easily.

Just as you allowed your coding processes to remain tentative until such time as you had a solid basis for confidence in a particular data grouping, you'll want to allow yourself various mechanisms for confirming the reasoning basis upon which you begin to identify patterns and relationships within the data. Although the term "validation" is sometimes used in the literature to allude to the idea of truth measures, what constitutes truth is a somewhat challenging proposition in interpretive description (as with most qualitative studies), especially when you are in the midst of data analysis. One technique that some qualitative researchers advocate is "member checks" (Erlandson, Harris, Skipper, & Allen, 1993), whereby you go back to your study participants to ascertain whether they will confirm having said what you think they said. In general, I would not recommend this, as it can lead to false confidence if they confirm what you thought, and potentially derail you from good analytic interpretations if they do not (Lincoln & Guba, 1985; Thorne & Darbyshire, 2005). In interpretive description, a researcher is not simply a vehicle through which study participants speak, but an interpretive instrument capable of making sense among cases to uncover insights that would not normally be accessible to you if you were only familiar with any single case. Therefore, although it is terribly important to ensure that you have your facts straight, depending on the nature of the study it may or may not be appropriate to assess whether the study participants themselves would agree with the interpretations you are drawing on the basis of the accounts they may have provided.

Expanding on Associations While the conventional "member check" may have limited utility, I believe that going back to the source of the data, either systematically or selectively, is often an extremely important step in transforming data into findings. When you bring your observations and initial tentative interpretations based upon them back to the study participants from which your insights derived, you are sharing with them not simply a reiteration of their own contributions, but rather a synthesis of what you have learned from many such encounters, and offering an opportunity to have them reflect on the extent to which it does or does not ring true to their experience. Using repeat interviews as a mechanism for confirmation, clarification, and elaboration on the essential relationships you are beginning to suspect within the overall data set is a powerful tool for helping you clarify what seems self-evident (but sometimes not articulated) to those involved, for surfacing the philosophizing they may have done about their situation, and for testing out the impact that giving the ideas some shape will have upon their understanding and experience. A similar effect can be achieved with strategic purposive sampling for new cases, shaping the interview strategies quite differently from the initial encounters by informing them with the evolving analysis. Ideally, this dialectic between the data collection and analysis occurs until you have formulated a compelling basis upon which to draw conclusions as to findings.

With member checking, you tend to feel you have done the right thing if everyone agrees with what you said you heard. With a more productive return to your sources, you are actually seeking that which challenges your thinking, pushes you further, and gives you more questions to ask yourself. It is these challenges that will allow you to avoid stopping at the obvious, to keep interrogating what you think you are finding, and to dig deep enough to generate findings that have real meaning and usefulness.

Testing Relationships As you move forward with your analysis, you will want to ask yourself "What ideas are starting to take shape such that I think they will have to have a place in my final analysis if it is to do justice to the research question?" This kind of question takes you back to the scaffolding supporting your original research question, including assumptions and expectations you may have brought into the study. When you challenge the relationships among data about which you are feeling increasingly confident against this backdrop, you step back from the immediacy of being immersed in data and allow yourself to see the emerging analysis within the context of that larger purpose for the study. In this manner, you make it easier to identify those elements of the emerging relationships that require "testing" or further challenge. This reflective step is quite helpful as you determine how you might go about engaging in that testing in order to effectively ground your eventual findings.

It is very exciting when the ideas you are forming about relationships begin to really take shape and form patterns. While it can be tempting to try to "nail them down" immediately, your note-making habit will allow you to document them for future reference while continuing to keep them in a state of suspension until you are well along the path of analysis. At this stage, you will be asking yourself such questions as "What pieces of the puzzle am I beginning to see?" and "What do they tell me about the puzzle as a whole?" By allowing your thinking to move back and forth between the parts and the whole, you'll increase your likelihood of detecting weaker relationships, identifying what to do about them, and deciding how you might work with them before they can become a viable part of the eventual whole you are building.

Capitalizing on Outliers Another set of questions you might pose as your analytic process unfolds includes, "What might I not be seeing?" If you assume that you cannot have captured all possible relevant variations, then your thinking allows you to probe questions like "What else might there be to see and how would I know that?" Although we usually fully intend to seek maximal variation within our study samples, we can't really know until we are fully immersed in the study what the entire set of truly relevant variables will include. Our initial purposive sampling strategy typically includes the demographic or conditional variables that we can predict from the literature might lead to variation within the experience. However, it is not until we have begun to formulate ideas about relationships among data that we can authentically discern the more relevant latent conceptual variables (Boychuk Duchscher & Morgan, 2004; Glaser, 2002). In some instances, once we've detected that we ought to see a case that meets certain conditions, we can locate that case and expand our data collection. In other instances, we can only theorize that cases fitting such conditions might exist.

I believe that it is important to ensure that the idea of what might have been found from cases not included in the study is built into the analytic process of an interpretive description study. Rather than claiming "saturation" (which has become a ubiquitous and somewhat arrogant assumption that one has tapped all relevant human variation (Caelli, Ray & Mill, 2003)), I encourage theorizing outliers and engaging in an imaginal exercise to shed light on what they might have contributed (McPherson & Thorne, 2006). In some instances, you can create virtual access to the outlying case through published literature reports or through recollections of "expert witnesses," including practicing clinicians who may have encountered rare instances in the course of their practice. Whether the outliers are available to you or not, merely thinking through what it is that they might have theoretically contributed to your evolving analysis can often be sufficient to ensure that you frame your findings in a manner that does not ignore predictable as well as rare but relevant variation.

Engaging the Critic Some of us have a sufficiently disciplined habit of mind that we are able to forcefully critique our own analysis even as we are fully immersed in it. Others may find that aspect of interpretive description excruciatingly difficult, and may devote considerable energy toward avoiding self-criticism or defending their position. However, if we deflect critique of our ongoing analysis, no matter how tempting, it will become difficult along the way to develop the kind of grounded confidence that one really depends upon to sustain the analysis through to conceptualization and writing up of findings as well as to the later elements of critically examining findings and considering their implications. Because inductive analysis relies on a part of the mind that feels generative rather than formally "analytic," scrupulously honest analysts can easily find themselves worrying that they are "making this up." In contrast, the researcher who is overly confident that there is only one story to tell may not have recognized his or her own role within the telling.

Although it is important to stay in control of the findings that you are building in articulating relationships among data, and to ensure that all aspects of the account are thoroughly grounded in a highly particularized manner, you can employ the external critic to great advantage within this process. By capitalizing on the tensions arising from the way that other people might read the same data, you paradoxically increase your sense of confidence by allowing yourself to understand and account for different perspectives. Sometimes it is useful to set up an actual or virtual "dialogue" between opposing perspectives on what the data reveal as a mechanism to exploit variations. Another technique you can experiment with involves going back to the literature, checking to see whether the "new insights" are really all that new, and challenging yourself with how certain authors or experts might see elements within your data quite differently. Asking what a particular expert might have said about the patterns you are seeing within the data can help you sort out the extent to which you may be relying on particular angles of vision and perhaps obscuring others as you begin to formulate the understandings that will best serve the research question, capitalize on the available data, and meet the ultimate purpose of your interpretive description research.

While data analysis is a complex and difficult challenge—one of those experiential aspects of life that you cannot truly appreciate until you have been immersed in it—it is important to remind yourself that it is entirely manageable and that there are countless strategies you can employ to ensure that it goes smoothly and well. A basic understanding of what it is that you are trying to accomplish and a good reading knowledge of a range of possible analytic techniques are foundational to the process. Even before you are ready to admit to yourself that you are in the analytic mode, your mind will begin to draw linkages between data bits and insert theoretical propositions upon what you hear and observe in the field. By attending to the cautions articulated here, and by ensuring that you employ technique to catalyze—rather than replace—thinking, you will find that the mind is the ultimate location for excellent inductive reasoning and conceptualization. Through iterative listening, observing, writing, thinking, listening, writing, thinking, and writing again, you will find that data begins to take shape, patterns and relationships form, and the possibility of meaningful and grounded conceptualizations draws closer. By engaging your mind, and having fun with the interpretive description analytic process, you make that goal your reality.

Conceptualizing Findings

Transforming Data

Identifying which data pieces are important, grouping and sorting them into patterns, and considering relationships between the pieces and patterns are all aspects of the complex inductive reasoning process through which you move closer to something that could constitute findings. In interpretive description, that which we consider "findings" is not simply reporting the first credible set of patterns that emerges from your sorting procedure. Rather, findings reflect an interpretive maneuver within which you consider what the pieces might mean, individually and in relation to one another, what various processes, structures, or schemes might illuminate about those relationships, and what order and sequence of presentation might most effectively lead the eventual reader toward a kind of knowing that was not possible prior to your study. In effect, you allow the reader to "know" something new about the phenomenon by virtue of the manner in which your rendering has both structured and sequenced it.

According to Wolcott, "interpretation is essentially a process and product of mulling" (1994, p. 287):

> When you emphasize description, you want your reader to see what you saw. When you emphasize analysis, you want your reader to know what you know. When you emphasize interpretation, you want your reader to understand what you think you yourself have understood. In different ratios, for different purposes, we try to accomplish all three (Wolcott, 1994, 412).

The decisions you make about what you aspire to and the groundings upon which you aim to achieve that end create a foundation for the manner in which your analytic process will transform data to become the eventual written report.

Envisioning a Conceptual Level

Sandelowski and Barroso's (2003a) taxonomy of qualitative findings provides a useful device for considering a range of possible outcomes using inductive techniques. At the most concrete end of the continuum of viable qualitative findings, they depict "topical survey" as an inventory of the topics that were covered by the study participants in response to the researcher's questions. In contrast, a "thematic summary" is a somewhat greater degree of transformation and abstraction than the topical survey, in that the research report reflects an ordered representation of initial groupings and patterns. In many instances, however, this kind of research report could have been generated on the basis of simple descriptive content analysis using predetermined themes and so, although it can permit reports of interesting data, it is not considered illustrative of the full potential that qualitative analysis can contribute. Moving to a level of higher abstraction, Sandelowski and Barroso describe the kind of study they portray as a "conceptual or thematic description." In this kind of report, thematic concepts exported from external sources or developed *in situ* from the data reveal latent patterns that have been discovered within the data through the application of the interpretive analytic process. Finally, the most fully integrated of qualitative analytic products yields what these authors have termed an "interpretive explanation." Such findings elucidate or clarify thematic linkages within a phenomenon in such a manner that they present it in an importantly new way. This new depiction is not simply an alternative linguistic or contextual variation on what has previously been understood, but takes the shape of a meaningful alternative claim that advances the field in some specific manner.

Using this taxonomy as a guide to articulating a range of qualitative findings, the object of interpretive description will typically be a thematic summary or a conceptual description. A report that reflects merely a topical survey will have fallen short of its intentions, and could have been generated using any standard content-analysis approach. At the other end of the spectrum, it is highly unlikely that a single, especially smaller, interpretive descriptive study will yield a fully matured and robust interpretive explanation, since the integrity and coherence of an entirely new conceptual angle on a phenomenon is dependent upon a highly rigorous and sophisticated approach to advanced theory testing within the analytic process itself. By understanding how these kinds of research products differ from the more typical products of an interpretive description study, you can orient your expectations within the parameters of what interpretive description permits, and avoid over-

or understating the findings that your analytic process allows you to formulate. Thus, instead of aiming to generate an exhaustive list of all topics that might possibly be linked to your phenomenon, or articulating a radically new metaphoric device with which to reference it, you will be able to keep your sights set on a thematic structure for showcasing the main elements of the phenomenon in relationship with one another, if not within a new conceptual or theoretical schema.

Working with Data Conceptually

When you can envision the form within which your eventual findings are likely to take shape, you can develop an increasingly refined set of mental and technical operations to advance your analysis toward that end. Although there is no shortcut to enthusiastic wrestling with your data, the intricate process of sense-making can begin early and continue throughout data collection and analysis such that the experienced researcher will have already considered and discarded or modified several conceptual approaches to working with the data before entering the final stages of formal data analysis. In the conceptual process, you become acutely aware of the important elements within your data set, the meta-messages that the final set of findings must convey to the reader if the report is to be true to the research, and the shortcomings of the study that will have to be acknowledged in the rendering of the final report. What you are therefore aiming for is a kind of conceptual structure within which to present and showcase the ideas that you are formulating, ideally one that will itself tell a key element of the larger story that demands telling.

The Cognitive Processes of Data Analysis Morse (1994b) has articulated a useful depiction of four sequential cognitive processes that are precursors to the kind of conceptualization that interpretive description requires. The first is *comprehending*, in which one learns everything one can about the setting or the experiences of the study participants. Morse believes that this process requires the capacity to hold judgments in abeyance and concentrate on passively absorbing everything remotely related to the situation being studied. From her perspective, this process begins with data collection, but continues through the data analysis process as coding and note-making are employed to generate an endless set of new questions that uncover deeper layers of understanding about the phenomenon.

The second cognitive process she names is *synthesizing*. In this process, you merge various instances or events to describe typical or composite patterns within the data. She sees this as a sifting process, in which the significant becomes distinguished from the insignificant and variations within the patterns become explainable. As she puts it, various factors "earn" their way into the data set as the synthesis evolves. Through synthesis, the researcher decontextualizes the processes from the individual instances of them, thereby extracting common features. Morse describes the act of synthesis as one of generating and manipulating speculation, verifying and falsifying elements within it, and selecting, revising, and discarding possibilities.

The third cognitive operation is *theorizing*, and developing "best guesses" about explanations. Within this process, additional questions can be asked of the data and considered on the basis of insights from other theoretical or empirical sources.

The final process for Morse is *recontextualizing*, a step within which the researcher articulates that which has been synthesized into a form that is applicable to other settings and contexts. This process brings the purely theoretical back to the practical, and permits a full appreciation for the implications of the newly generated knowledge.

Morse's taxonomy of cognitive operations is helpful in understanding what is involved in the rigorous conceptual work that shapes the eventual findings. Her depiction clearly emphasizes that it is the researcher, and not the recipe, that is driving the interpretive process. However, despite the broad sequential nature of the cognitive operations outlined in this taxonomy, the actual experience of interpretive description does tend to feel much more iterative than sequential. What a schema such as Morse's provides, though, is a way of ensuring that you are mobilizing a shifting blend of cognitive operations as the analytic process moves from early exploration through to a coherent conceptual structure. It may not serve as a specific guide to "what's next," but will help you monitor the time and energy you are devoting to the various elements within the analytic process. New researchers typically get bogged down in comprehension (one can never fully know everything after all) or move too quickly into synthesis on the basis of assumptions that their comprehension is complete. The mental attitudes Morse proposes can be helpful in steering us back on course if we find ourselves off target.

The Mechanics of Advancing Conceptual Analysis As you work your data from pieces and parts into patterns and relationships and toward more integrated conceptual claims and interpretations, you begin to appreciate the value of tapping a range of strategies for discovering which analytic options will be possible on the basis of your particular data set. In many ways, this is like having a large set of building blocks, and experimenting with the different ways their form and structure enable and constrain what you are capable of constructing.

An important angle to keep firmly in mind is that your entire design and research approach are predicated on the value of inductive knowledge development. What you will want to avoid is moving too quickly in your analytic process into major categories (such as events or processes) and then being tempted to fill in the bits in your ongoing data collection. Such an intellectual process reverses your logic into a deductive approach, which of course will become circular and self-defeating because you did not design the kind of study that would justify that form of reasoning. Thus, always guarding against the demon of premature closure no matter how eager you are for project completion, it can be important to repeatedly return to reading your raw data and jotting down new ways of thinking about it into the "blank pages" of your notebook as a device to encourage you to begin the analytic thought process afresh.

If your first few attempts yield similar patterns, it is likely that you have not yet allowed your mind to fully explore alternative ways of depicting structure. You may find, on reflection, that you are having difficulty letting go of your preconceptions or prior allegiances about the topic. As a special caution, this issue becomes particularly problematic where the field is dominated by a particularly influential thinker—such as Goffman (1968) on the topic of stigma in illness—or where your research supervisor has staked a claim upon a particular way of conceptualizing the topic. If, on honest reflection, you really don't have options beyond the existing theories, you might consider simply using your inquiry as an explicit mechanism for advancing them, and avoid pretense that your findings have derived from an original inductive analytic approach. If, on the other hand, such an exercise produces wildly diverse iterations, you have an excellent basis from which to interrogate one against another, asking such questions as "What will this structure illuminate that this other will not?" and "What does it mean that certain elements are more prominent in this scheme than in the other?" This step will allow you to engage in a rigorous process of keeping both (or all) possibilities in play as long as comparing and contrasting them in this way continues to give way to new insights.

Rather than beginning with major categories before you establish the smaller ones, try to stay deep within your data set as you begin to label and link the various elements. While you are not initially seeking formal relationships, you may well find that it is natural to begin by articulating a range of possible associations between elements. Each new relationship you propose will allow you to raise further questions that will advance your appreciation for the possibilities inherent in the data set. As the pieces grow and become more firmly established in your mind as essential elements within your overall conceptual structure, you can risk more formal labeling. However, as with premature coding, it is useful to keep reminding yourself that the label you have designated for each set of similar ideas or themes is merely a device for organizing your thinking and has not become a fixed reality of any kind. Remember that labels are mental devices by which we can sort and retrieve information, and that they can mislead if taken overly literally. Being willing to suspend committing to a final nomenclature for the parts of your overall puzzle until quite late in the analytic phase will allow you to exploit new angles of interpretation that present themselves throughout the process.

As the conceptual whole of your interpretive description begins to build, it does become important to work out options for organizing the various pieces into coherent groupings and lists. At this stage, it is essential to "try out" a range of organizational options so that you can begin to understand the implications of each for your write-up, for the form of the final findings, and for what you will be able to do with the findings once they have been articulated. You might ask yourself questions like "What happens if I group what I have in this way versus this other?" or "In what way are these groupings different, and why would that matter?" What you are seeking here is an understanding of the logic model that will guide the structuring of your report of findings from a particular beginning to a particular end. The ingredients of the story and the sequence within which they are presented will depend upon your capacity to know where to begin and how you intend to conclude. You might consider various options such as moving within your material from superficial to deep, simple to complex, manifest to underlying, past to present, consequential to central. In general, an overall structure to the material you will be considering becomes an important element of the conceptualization, and will be a fundamental requisite to the successfully executed write-up.

The Art and Science of Conceptualizing

A well-integrated piece of interpretive description not only generates a coherent report that depicts and links common elements of a clinical phenomenon, but it also generates a mental heuristic that makes that new understanding accessible to the practitioner target audience

---

TEXT BOX 9.1

Adjusting to Chronic Illness

Rayman and Ellison used interpretive description to better understand the day-by-day reality of women learning intensive control for managing type 2 diabetes. Because this period of illness adjustment has been described as one of chaos and disruption, they sought an understanding that might lead to interventions to positively influence disease management and improve ultimate outcomes. Within their sample of women, they documented three distinct patterns of response. Some women were engaged in disease management and adapting, some were engaged and struggling, and a few were what they categorized as "pre-engaged." The struggles the researchers documented included those associated with self, food, and relationships. This analysis allowed the authors to reflect on the complexity of the social context and the multilayered experience within which these women were immersed. They were able to track patterns in the dynamics that women experienced through these early months of adjustment. Their findings confirm the dramatic changes that individuals newly diagnosed with diabetes must make to their preferences, habits, roles, and lifestyle, and how important it is that they receive transitional support from health care providers who understand what they are going through.

Raymans, K. M. & Ellison, G.C. (2004). Home alone: The experience of women with type 2 diabetes who are new to intensive control. *Health Care for Women International, 25*, 900–915.

(Thorne, Reimer Kirkham et al., 2004). The ideal might be described as a research report that makes visible and accessible the clinical wisdom of a passionate and thoughtful expert practitioner for whom a similar understanding had been acquired through extensive pattern recognition and reflective practice observations. While theory may play some role in assisting you to come up with such heuristics, the ultimate purpose is not theorizing but rather illuminating insight. Thus the kind of conceptual claim that you are striving toward is unlikely to be highly abstract, original, or metaphoric, but is one that will powerfully capture the important elements within the clinical phenomenon in a manner that can be grasped, appreciated and remembered in the applied context. Whether such a conceptualization is achievable within your particular study is something you may not be able to predict until you have worked through the analytic process, and so it is often wise to allow yourself some leeway in determining the ultimate form of your findings until you have established your options. If, for example, a conceptual description is just beyond your reach, then you might do better to represent your findings in the form of a thematic summary rather than stretching credibility by suggesting a coherence you cannot reasonably justify.

The Nature of Concepts

Concepts are mental devices for organizing ideas so that we can communicate them to one another and build complex bodies of knowledge. They are the foundational building blocks of human organization, and allow us to transform the vast complexity of experience and thought into controllable pieces such that we can manage in the world. The capacity to conceptualize has been described as that which makes us uniquely human, and that which allows us to handle knowledge in the manner that we do. We are surrounded by concepts, and they shape the vast majority of what we experience as well as our capacity to reason. We know that they are fluid and socially constructed, and yet they can be remarkably stable and persistent where they seem to fit some important human purpose.

Although we embrace concepts continuously as part of our shared human experience, they do seem to get us into trouble when we try to manipulate them for the purpose of knowledge development. We have very few mechanisms for communicating ideas without relying upon shared conceptual knowledge, and yet our dependence upon concepts can mislead us into thinking we "know" that which has been presented in conceptual form. For this reason, many scholars, including qualitative researchers, strive toward creating new concepts that will compete with the old as a mechanism for advancing new knowledge.

An example from the health domain may illustrate. For many years, the concept "noncompliance" was routinely used to reference the idea that some patients fail to follow the advice of their physician with regard to a medical treatment or health behavior recommendation. Because that concept was understood to imply that the physician had all the right answers and the patient's role was to passively follow orders, many health scientists and clinicians began to advocate for an alternative concept—"adherence." While this was a well-intended move, simply changing the vocabulary without tackling the underlying values had very little effect on the original problem, and essentially diverted the attention that might have been put toward solving it into debating the relative merits of the two linguistic options. In this instance,

TEXT BOX 9.2

Healing from Troubled Childhood

Henderson and Jackson took an interpretive descriptive approach to their study of how vulnerable young women understand the impact of difficult life circumstances on their current state of health and well-being. The "at risk" girls who participated in focus groups had had troubled childhoods; many experienced substance abuse and violence. Although most had current involvement with both the courts and the health care system, their complex backgrounds made it difficult for them to obtain help or support within conventional service settings. Comparing themes among the stories of these girls, Henderson and Jackson bring the complexity to life, and allow an outsider to understand the anger, frustration, and despair that characterize their experience. The experiential perspectives of the disjuncture between what the health care system provides and what these girls thought they needed make it understandable that many felt their best guarantee of support was through being picked up and jailed. These findings form a basis upon which the authors advocate for a concept of restorative health to match the restorative justice that has recently been popularized as a humane approach to complex socio-criminal problems.

Henderson, A.D., & Jackson, M. (2004). Restorative health: Lessening the impact of previous abuse and violence in the lives of vulnerable girls. *Health Care for Women International, 25,* 794–812.

revising the concept label did nothing to change the concept, and the embedded structural problem remained quite persistent until an entirely new way of thinking about the phenomenon emerged, complete with its own lexicon. In the world of chronic illness care, the idea of "self-care decision making" is not only being articulated but also politically advanced, as a revolutionary new approach to thinking about and delivering services. What this example illustrates is that merely fiddling with the packaging of an idea is rarely sufficient to enact any meaningful result in knowledge development, while finding an original conceptual approach that forces rethinking an old problem may be quite powerful.

In the medical world, many concepts are known by the name of the originator (Colles' fracture, Heimlich maneuver, Alzheimer's disease). In the social and health care context, the concepts that seem most likely to be understood and taken up in a meaningful way are those that adapt "common" language to clearly communicate a new intent. Thus "patient rights," "consumer advocacy," "informed consent" are the kinds of ideas that develop around a conceptual grounding, allowing us to locate the conversation we are in, to discern the claims that are being made about the concept, and to understand what is being suggested in terms of the relationships that are being proposed between it and other concepts. Interpretive description has the potential to generate new conceptualizations, or to inform refinements on the attributes and operational elements we understand in relation to existing concepts. In my own early work with a colleague, we were lucky enough to generate the concept "guarded alliance" to refer to the reconstructed but vigilant form of trust that chronically ill people allowed themselves to form with their professional health care providers (Thorne & Robinson, 1989). Although the informing research was conducted before we were referring to the approach as "interpretive description," it was a clear instance of the kind of conceptual contribution that interpretive description seeks to generate. As an idea, it helps clinicians understand that chronically ill patients who maintain an element of mistrust in their relationships with clinicians are likely protecting themselves against predictable experiences and demonstrating a healthy responsibility for their own well-being. With that idea in mind, you are less likely to be irritated by the scrutiny of your patients and more likely to find ways to celebrate their active agency.

The problem with concepts is that we don't actually control them, but rather they are (or are not) taken up as meaningful and useful for some purpose, and tend to take on a life of their own. When an idea finds a receptive audience, it can become embedded in the social fabric like wildfire. Consider, for example, the recent enthusiasm for "environmental sustainability," an important idea that was always there, but now seems top of mind in political life and public discourse. The uptake of the concept may well have been facilitated by various influential people and events, but it is also an idea for which society at large was remarkably receptive.

Ownership of concepts—the right to define them and articulate their properties and attributes—is a hotly contested arena. Because they are an important commodity in shaping our collective lives, there is much to be gained by trying to manipulate what is or is not included within the concept, and which conceptual relationships will be permitted. Although we scientists spend a lot of our intellectual effort advancing and attempting to control concepts, it is not we who get to determine the impact, but rather this becomes a product of audience reaction. Thus understanding something of the nature of concepts and the machinations of conceptual knowledge can help you avoid getting caught in the absurdities of definitional wars and instead keep you focused on the larger objective toward which conceptual knowledge is directed. In general, we are conducting research because we believe something ought to be understood or handled differently. Whether the invention of an original conceptual label for that phenomenon will or will not effect that change is something we all ought to consider before directing all of our interpretive description aspirations toward conceptual solutions.

Conceptualizing Through Thematic Description

Armed with a healthy reverence for the complexities inherent not only in generating conceptually integrated findings but also doing something with them once you have developed them, you may find yourself more appreciative of the usefulness of an artfully conducted thematic summary. Certainly, as an appropriate product of an interpretive description, the thematic summary can offer all the advantages of the conceptual description without the risk of deluding yourself as to the import and originality of your contribution to knowledge.

A good thematic description is distinguished from the topical summary by virtue of the extent to which the organizing structure within which it is presented itself becomes part of the new conceptualization. Without making claims to the invention of new concepts, the thematic summary can "show" the audience how elements within the larger phenomenon can be ordered and organized to reveal aspects that would have been obscured through any other presentation framework. Thus, the organizing structure within which such a research product is presented is a result of enlightened conceptualizing without setting out to knock down existing concepts or invent new ones.

The core ingredients of conceptualizing are ideas, and the mechanisms with which we work with them are words and signifiers. Thus, as the analytic process evolves, we move from rudimentary groupings reflecting similarities and differences within the data ("Category A" data, for example), toward conceptual labels with the potential to shape the accessibility of those ideas to the eventual reader. It is important to recognize that the labels with which we categorize and handle patterns and relationships within our data set are conveyers of conceptual meaning. Thus, finding ways to further the larger understanding

---

TEXT BOX 9.3

Being Radioactive

Stajduhar and colleagues used an interpretive description approach to document the experience that patients with thyroid cancer have as a result of a highly radioactive treatment requiring strict isolation during hospitalization. What interviews with these patients revealed was that these patients were overwhelmed by the enormity of having a cancer diagnosis, and in this context felt profoundly affected by the social and physical isolation that their treatment necessitated. They found the treatment safety precautions equally overwhelming, and many conducted their own research to ensure that they understood their circumstances as well as possible. At the same time, they worried that they were unprepared for what it would entail, and were highly anxious about any inconsistent messages they received about such matters as nutritional restrictions and the handling of personal items exposed to radiation. By documenting common patterns and themes in the experience of this particular group of patients, Stajduhar and colleagues were able to generate some immediate recommendations to ensure optimal care contexts for these patients.

Stajduhar, K. I., Neithercut, J., Chu, E., Pham, P., Rodhe, J., Sicotte, A., & Young, K. (2000). Thyroid cancer: Patients' experiences of receiving iodine-131 therapy. *Oncology Nursing Forum, 27*(8), 1213–1218.

---

through the syntax of our thematic organizing structure becomes an important way to advance knowledge. By recognizing this process as a conceptual process, and not simply a poetic or catchy set of phrases or thematic subheadings, we elevate thematic summary to a more meaningful and coherent position.

To illustrate, in a study of oral health care within long-term-care residential facilities, we interviewed and conducted participant observation to try to develop knowledge about how such services worked. In our written report, we chose not to organize our findings according to effective versus ineffective approaches or by specific elements within the service (dental care, everyday hygiene support). Instead we articulated overarching conceptual structures that seemed to interact to shape the context within which each element became more or less effective (Thorne, Kazanjian, & MacEntee, 2001). In our report, organizing our thematic observations and interpretations using "programmatic strategies" and "organizational culture" as intersecting variables allowed us to advance a conceptual understanding that a variable like oral health care was sufficiently contextually and relationally embedded that the actual mechanism of oral health service delivery was of relative unimportance. Had we attempted to convey these insights in the form of a new concept label or metaphoric representation, we might have completely lost our audience. Instead, from what we have heard, our findings created a basis upon which various care facilities could justify a range of approaches toward meeting their larger care objectives—whether or not they explicitly targeted oral health.

What you are aiming for in your interpretive description, whether through conceptual or thematic approaches, is a means for organizing and presenting findings such that something below surface meaning—beyond the self-evident—can be explored and elucidated. You want to show evidence of alternative explanations you have considered, and you want to ensure that the analytic forms or metaphors that emerge as the infrastructure for presenting your findings are selected on the basis of their capacity to convey an appreciation for the context of the phenomenon, not simply for their effectiveness in crafting a good story out of the data.

Interpretive description is always a meaning-making activity, directed at a particular kind of audience (such as clinicians) toward the purpose of rendering a new, enriched, or expanded way of making sense of some problem or issue. Although it does not necessarily contain normative components—for there are times when excellent description is sufficient in itself—in many instances an interpretive description product does reflect assumptions about what an ideal future might look like, which is a logical outgrowth of the problem that drives it (patients with fewer pain problems, newly diagnosed patients with less emotional distress, and so on). In order to be of excellent quality, it must retain an integrity to that sense of direction throughout the process and in the product of the research, such that what it claims to have generated is consistent with the steps that comprised the generation. Interpretive description fails to achieve its potential if it does not extend understanding beyond what was there before. A new organizing structure, or new conceptual labels, in and of themselves do nothing for advancing knowledge (and arguably can contribute to the collective confusion). When those organizing structures reveal new possibilities in the relationship between subjective experience and conceptual knowledge, they will have achieved their essential purpose.

Drawing Analysis to Conclusion

Through rigorous processes and thoughtful iterative analysis and synthesis, you eventually arrive at your conceptual or thematic apex. With any luck, you'll be sufficiently confident of one way of conceptualizing your findings in comparison to all other possible options that you can begin to formalize the findings report. By understanding the tale you want to tell, you'll provide yourself with the explicit blueprint for which pieces and parts will need to be brought into the mix and lined up in a particular sequence so that you can lead a reader, not necessarily down the identical path you followed, but through to the same general conclusion.

It is sometimes difficult, especially for the inexperienced, to read the signals accurately as to whether you have arrived at a sufficiently strong analytic foundation to be able to write up the findings. What you are seeking is the capacity to use your conceptual or thematic structure in such a manner that it guides your decisions as you sequence material and select which angles to emphasize and what illustrations to profile. You want your organizing structure to answer such questions as "What belongs where?", "How much detail is needed?" and "Which aspects of the issue at hand should I document and how do I most effectively present them?" As a rule of thumb, your analysis has reached an appropriate conclusion when you can not only articulately and credibly generate a detailed "table of contents" depicting the major headings and minor subheadings that will shape your account of the findings, but also argue (or write) a convincing introduction to the findings that explains why the material is organized in the manner that it is and by what logic the reader will be helped to access it. When you have accomplished this step effectively, it becomes apparent which elements of your raw data will be relevant, where and how, and to what use they will be put. With the outline of the portrait making explicit the features it will include, you are ready to begin to paint the picture.

CHAPTER TEN

Writing Findings

Setting the Stage

Beginning to write your findings is among the most exciting and daunting steps in an interpretive description project. It is a stage you have imagined from the beginning—envisioning brilliant textual excerpts framed by elegant narrative and spiraling into breathtakingly novel and compelling conclusions. Needless to say, although writing the findings is quite different from the drudgery of writing up a literature review or the hard slogging of articulating the methodological approach, it does not typically "flow" in the manner that we might have imagined. There is an art to the writing that requires both patience and discipline, and you may make several false starts before you find the approach that will work for you and serve the demands of your particular research project.

Judging Your Readiness

Readiness to write is among the difficult judgments that a newer researcher has to make, and it is made all the more difficult by our human differences relative to any disciplined process. As was suggested in the previous chapter, it is always preferable to wait until you can defend the organizational structure that derives from your conceptualization of the phenomenon before you begin the writing process. However, many writers don't quite realize they haven't fully grasped the implications of that structure until they actually begin to write it. So thinking about the writing and conceptualizing stages as yet another iterative process can be helpful in avoiding discouragement.

Sometimes you'll have the advantage of an audience to which you can present your tentative findings prior to writing them. Many researchers create self-imposed deadlines by submitting abstracts to conferences or offering to share their findings before they are fully solidified. You can turn this to good advantage if you test out an organizing structure that you can envision and defend, and you can also invite explicit critique into the aspects of the whole that seemed not to "hang together."

Readiness to write is another element of research that is strongly influenced by your basic characterological makeup. Some of us are naturally more hesitant, recognizing that we'll never have all of the answers, and others leap ahead blissfully confident that it will all come together nicely. Knowing your own characteristic style, and ensuring that it works for you instead of against you, is central to your maturity as a researcher. For neophytes, colleagues and supervisors can often be your best source of guidance as to whether you are the kind of person who needs to be pushed or restrained in order to achieve the optimal balance for your project.

Deciding on Structure

There are two basic ways to present interpretive description findings, and which you choose will typically depend on the balance you have achieved between description and interpretation in conceptualizing your findings. The first is to organize the findings within an overarching conceptual claim, the elements of which become the organizing structure for the pieces required in order to understand the whole. The second is to recognize that, if you don't have a conceptual argument of sufficient potency to become the findings, you will need to set up a sequenced organizing framework that will not be the story in and of itself but will allow you to tell the story. Knowing which kind of report you are aiming for becomes important in generating the detailed roadmap for writing that you will need to keep you honest.

Understanding the nature of that overall structure will also guide you in your decisions as to what headings and subheadings you will be working with in order to bring your findings to life. If your powerful message is the larger conceptual one, then the sequence and syntax of the various headings must communicate that clearly and articulately. If the organizing structure is the platform upon which the true findings will be showcased, then it can be a mistake to be overly flowery or metaphoric in your headings, as those props will compete for attention with the central characters. As Sandelowski puts it, you need to understand whether your organizing structure ought to be emphasizing "character, scene, or plot" (1998, p. 377). As an aside, I'd also suggest that understanding the nature of your overall structure should also guide you in the eventual selection of the title for your work. Some very good studies have been disregarded for having identified themselves with a level of conceptual abstraction that they could not sustain internally. So what you are seeking is a match between the form of the findings and the conceptual level implied in the title.

I would not recommend that anyone begin writing interpretive description findings without a clearly articulated outline. For those who think best in concept maps, the form of that outline may be a visual representation (such as bubbles and arrows or concentric circles). However, for most of us, there is no better structuring system than the good old fashioned table of contents outline format. Given that (in most instances) you will likely have to write the chapter in word sequences that require one sentence before another, paragraphs in some logical order, a beginning, middle, and an end, it does make sense to meticulously organize that sequential order before trying to enact it.

In general, perhaps because of the limits and peculiarities of our human minds as they try to grasp complex concepts, a set of findings tends to be most typically organized into a "handful" of major groupings (such as four ways of responding, six distinct kinds of experience, five steps in a process, or three overall patterns of interaction). If you find you have too many or two few "major" groupings, you may want to ask yourself whether you have fully concluded your conceptual process, or whether there are additional structural alternatives you might still consider. Many neophyte researchers find themselves wanting to argue that they can't possibly break up what is a "whole" experience into component parts, and therefore resist attempts to articulate structural groupings. While we might sympathize with the sentiment that human experience is holistic in nature, that particular argument fails to fly when it comes to writing a research report. You actually do need to order and organize parts of a whole in order to build a sequential argument that will allow your reader to come to the understanding you intend. No matter how passionately you argue that your particular phenomenon defies structural definition, your reader still needs to grasp the relevant bits in order to accept what you conclude as a whole. So, thoughtful decisions as to how you will structure the parts of your findings for presentation is an essential element in effectively conveying your newfound insights in written form.

When you have in your mind the appropriate set of component parts—those major headings that will form the organizing structure for your findings write-up—you will need to name them. It is important to recognize that, whatever form or style of label you choose, they will have to relate to one another (reflect the same grammatical style, a similar level of abstraction, a parallel kind of conceptualization) and they will have to have some kind of logical sequence. There will always be a first section, then a second, and so on, and your decision as to this sequence should never be arbitrary. It is useful to think of yourself as telling a story, and needing to find a logic with which to justify what is the best place to begin, what will happen along the way, and how it will all end. The table of contents style of writing blueprint remains the trustworthy companion to most skilled writers because it lays bare the groupings, allows you to "massage" the labels by which you will represent them, and forces you to come to grips with the sequence with which they will be addressed within the writing. From this comes the insight to know just how each section ought to be written, how much depth and detail should be included, and which ideas will be best left for later. A structure that ultimately supports your understanding of the intricate interrelationship between each of the tiny component parts within the written product is the one that will differentiate excellent writing—and a good read—from that which doesn't quite meet the mark.

Although some research write-ups may not appear to require formal structure beyond major groupings (the page restrictions of many scholarly journals precluding excessive use of subheadings), longer reports (such as dissertations or monographs) will most certainly require an overt organizing framework that includes more than one layer of structure. And whether the subheadings actually appear in the eventual written text, it is important to extend the planning exercise as far into the structural detail as possible. When the major groupings are articulated in a form and sequence that will serve the whole, each must be considered for its own internal structure. Each will have its own component parts, and they too should be sequenced and labeled (the label being less essential if you don't intend to use subheadings, but equally integral to the writing blueprint nevertheless).

As a test for the effectiveness of your writing outline, it can be instructive to go back to your data before you begin to write. As you review and reread text, you will be asking yourself whether you can distinguish between that which is central to the argument you will be building, that which is contextual, and that which is sufficiently peripheral or distracting that it will not find its way into the final text. Where you encounter bits (such as case exemplars of a key element) that you know will have to be in the final write-up, can you quickly determine where they must be located within the whole in order to attain the best effect? It is the capacity of your structural framework to organize you in the process of writing that will ultimately determine its ability to inform your reader.

Determining a Writing Style

Writing well is a fundamental competency within all qualitative research (Wolcott, 1990). We have all read a great deal of research reporting by the time we come to do it ourselves, and typically will have formulated some impressions of what our own findings write-up will look like. We may have a favorite author whose style of writing we intend to emulate, or a voice within our head that has been pressing for expression. It is wise to pay attention to those preferences and impressions as they are likely to find expression even when we aren't explicitly giving them permission. For most of us, writing involves a cacophony of urgent voices all wanting to find their way onto the page in some manner or other, and requiring some kind of choirmaster to bring them all into harmony. If you ignore them, they tend to sneak in on their own in a less controllable manner than if you befriend them, so self-knowledge becomes an important part of managing your writing process.

Writing an interpretive description allows you to be somewhat more creative in your writing than your research proposal will have permitted, and yet finding the balance between scholarship and creativity can be frustratingly complex. When you allow your creativity to flow with excess profusion, perhaps waxing poetical or invoking the heights of passion in your writing, you jeopardize your ability to sustain credibility. Conversely, if you write up your findings in a dry and technical manner, very little is likely to excite your reader sufficiently to grasp the importance of your message. Because the purpose of your study, in most instances, will be to have illuminated certain elements of human subjective experience for the purpose of expanding the capacity of a practice discipline to solve problems, you do want to find approaches within your writing that will showcase the message and bring it to the attention of the intended audience. No single writing style can possibly serve all of the various projects that might warrant interpretive description (Sandelowski, 1998).

The form of your research report will most likely include some combination of narrative and exemplars from your data set. Thinking through how you will tackle this, and coming up with an approach that will effectively serve your needs does require some planning. It goes without saying that data do not "speak for themselves." We have all heard presentations by neophyte researchers who have abdicated their role and responsibility as researchers and chosen instead to share with us snippets of text—verbatim quotes from their favorite study participants and so on. If data spoke for themselves, research would be redundant, and we would not have to bother with method (Thorne & Darbyshire, 2005). Just as a journalist has a clear agenda in choosing certain persons to interview, selecting quick phrases to quote, and placing the report within a particular context, research is also strongly associated with a particular social role, process, and expected product. The data you have harvested and conceptualized are privileged materials, obtained on the basis of a social trust as to how they ought to be used and within the context of a particular academic or clinical community. It is your obligation to continue to steer the process through to its logical conclusion, and to use those precious data thoughtfully and defensibly in making what will be represented as empirical claims. So regardless of your sentimental attachment to your study participants (and all qualitative researchers feel that!), the report of findings will be the product of your logic, grounded in the data you have co-constructed, and presented to the audience you intend to enrich with your contribution to knowledge. You will draw strategically upon excerpts of the data to illustrate the points you are making, but it will be you who is deciding which points deserve a place in the written report and why.

When you have accepted the mantle of responsibility for the structure and process of the research report, you come to appreciate that your logical reasoning becomes the thread of argument that must contain the entire presentation. You have to know where you are going and why, how to signal your reader as to where you are in the journey, when you have come to a transition point, and when you are nearing the end. You will generate the narrative that glues the entire write-up together and provides the fabric within which the textual excerpts, verbatim quotes, and case examples become the decoration. For this reason, it is essential to (at least theoretically if not literally) separate out the narrative from the illustrative elements to your writing. While the final report may reflect a blend of you speaking and your study participants echoing your statements in their own unique voices, it is usually best to begin by writing the narrative and then later weaving in the examples. This way, you allow yourself to "see" the flow of logic, stay in control of your flow of ideas, paragraph structure, and linkages, and really position those examples, when they do find their way in, to best advantage. I often encourage graduate students to put their data bits aside temporarily and write the narrative first. This allows for a really thorough development of the whole, tests out the logic model you have constructed, and frames the entire written report convincingly.

It turns out not to be too difficult to go back then, to sort through and organize the marvelous examples you intend to include, and to massage them into the narrative at the appropriate juncture. What you'll typically find is that you have far more wonderful examples than you can appropriately accommodate, and so you'll need to decide which best serve the argument. More about that later.

It tends to be a terrible idea to begin the other way around—starting with collections of examples and trying to line them up into a coherent argument after the fact. In most instances, the astute reader can see evidence of that in the research report, and you might place yourself at risk for what Sandelowski and Barroso (2003a) would term a "no findings" study. Seasoned researchers may well be able to combine writing narrative with selecting examples in an initial draft, but for many who are newer at the exercise, it will be well worth separating those two distinct intellectual processes so that you can achieve some clarity of purpose with each.

Engaging in the Process

Finding Your Writer's Voice

A major challenge that many researchers confront when they finally sit down to begin writing is deciding the "voice" with which they will write. Beyond fairly straightforward decisions as to whether you'll permit first person (the alternative being to reference yourself as "the researcher"), you will be trying to find the writing tone and form that will authentically represent your motivation, do justice to your findings, and "speak to" your eventual reader. Your sentence structure, the words you choose, and the manner in which you make explicit the logical flow of your thinking are all elements of the way you interact with that reader and convey what will be read as credible or not. Thus your writing tone becomes a significant part of your responsibility in leading your project toward its successful conclusion. Being overly flippant, judgmental, arrogant, emotional, or self-absorbed can all be the kiss of death to your eventual effectiveness. So you are trying to convey something of yourself, your process, and your reasoning without highjacking your project.

Although the mind of the researcher is an integral element in the conduct of an interpretive description study, repeated reminders of that within the written report tend to distract the reader from confidence in the ultimate product. Constantly referencing what "my participants told me" tends to make the report just a bit too precious to be believable; instead, you will want to be using yourself as an instrument of the study rather than its primary focus. While it is your logic that will direct the structure and process of the narrative, you might keep your personhood at a discreet distance backstage, only allowing yourself to peek out temporarily where there is some aspect of the narrative, such as a particular contextual insight, that simply cannot be told in any other way.

Effective writing tends to be fairly simple and straightforward in structure and relatively accessible in its terminological choices. There can be a great temptation as you are seeking entrance to a new scholarly community to effect language and writing structure that seem more sophisticated, worldly, and difficult than what you have previously used. As Sandelowski reminds us,

> Whereas quantitative researchers may turn off their readers with jargon high on statistical, but low on clinical significance, qualitative researchers may offend with turgid prose, seemingly endless lists of unlinked codes and categories, dangling participles, and dizzying arrays of multiply hyphenated and, sometimes, nonexistent words that convey nothing more than the writer's willingness (albeit unintended) to destroy the English language (1998, p. 375).

Saying things in a more complex manner than is necessary and using obscure language merely obfuscates your purpose and tends to make your reader suspect thesaurus addiction rather than cleverness. The point of your research write-up is to excite the intelligence and imagination of your reader toward better understandings of a phenomenon you thought sufficiently important to warrant the effort of a research study. And so a writing voice that will be effective toward that purpose, one that appears to effortlessly guide your reader along a path of logic and insight whose outcome is the conceptual knowledge you have attained, is the kind of voice toward which you ought to be aiming. Once you have the basics of style and structure mastered, it is most certainly possible to dress it up a bit with your own particular brand of flourish, but do ensure that you are building creativity upon a solid foundation of good writing. If you look carefully at the writing of the scholars you consider your best virtual role models, including those who seem exemplars of "beautiful rendering" (Sandelowski, 1994a), you will notice that underlying their distinctive styles is mastery of the basic tenets of grammar and composition.

Strategizing Examples

As you think back to the purpose of interpretive description, you'll recall that it is not simply to uncover marvelous stories of human experience (for any qualitative method or good storyteller can accomplish that), but primarily to generate a species of knowledge that captures commonalities within human subjective experience at the same time as it allows us to think about individual variation. We develop general knowledge, not because it represents truth, but because it allows us to grasp and communicate about patterns within human behavior more effectively, and allows us to make better informed decisions about the individual cases that we will encounter professionally. This principle becomes important in the selection and articulation of the examples that you will use to illustrate the narrative argument you are building in your findings write-up, and will differentiate the products of interpretive description from those of some other qualitative research methods.

The point of using examples in your findings report is never to "prove" your claims. While judicious reference to data examples provides some assurance that the claims you make are grounded in the data, the reader essentially has to take much of what you say on faith, since there is no way of truly auditing all that you have done, seen, or heard in the course of your research. Further, even if you were to furnish multiple examples of a particular phenomenon, your sampling strategy prevents you from making the kinds of claims that numeric data imply in a manner that your reader will find justifiable (Sandelowski, 2001). Similarly, although it can support your argument to mention prevalence patterns within your particular sample, "always" and "never" are unlikely conclusions within the context of this kind of study.

You are, however, likely to want to help readers navigate between the kinds of instances that the examples within your data illustrate, whether that be a particularly extreme case of a thing or its prototypical exemplar. If you understand your purpose to be both illumination of commonalities and elaboration of some of the kinds of variations that you have observed within your data set, then your choice and presentation of examples will clearly position each within a part of your overall argument. In many instances, researchers begin with describing the common elements, perhaps selectively inserting illustrative quotations or anecdotes chosen to reveal central properties within them, and then proceed to demonstrating some of the kinds of variations that the data set has included. The manner in which you present model examples, contrasting examples, and "outliers" reflects your appreciation for the role each is playing in building the larger portrait of the phenomenon under study, rendering it both understandable through structure and complex through variation. You need to make this clear to your reader, so that the extreme variation is not misunderstood as common, and vice versa.

The best examples will typically be those that not only show the point you are making, but also do so in some utterly human and interesting manner. However, you will need to be careful that you don't overly rely on any one particular study participant, especially if that participant might be distinguishable to the reader by virtue of expression style or context. Whether you present them verbatim or paraphrase them will largely depend on how effectively the actual words and expressions will have captured the meaning you intend to illustrate. People typically do not express orally what translates easily onto the written page. You might know what someone "said," but find there is no specific sentence or paragraph in which that idea was neatly conveyed. In general, use just the amount of illustrative material that you need to make the specific point you are presenting. Too much detail raises additional questions in the mind of the reader and can derail you from the specific point about which you are trying to convince the reader. Where the words themselves are awkward, disjointed, or trail off, you may find that paraphrasing (reporting that someone said something instead of quoting the exact words) may be more appropriate. Unless you build in a great deal of context, your reader will not be attached to the personalities of your study participants in the way that you likely are. And so you are trying to be coolly objective in choosing the material and exemplars that best illustrate your findings, not those that democratically represent your original sample or your experience gathering data. Finally, do remember that the transformation between spoken word and written text requires that someone impose punctuation and sentence structure upon it. The reader needs to "hear" it in a structure that is intelligible, and it is your job to render it into that form.

Making the Audit Trail Accessible

Because the procedural elements involved in generating an excellent inductive analysis are quite difficult to capture linguistically within a written report, you'll need to ensure that you have provided sufficient guidance for the reader to distinguish between that which you are describing and that which you are interpreting. In some instances, you may find it appropriate to be explicit about your interpretive approach, but in most cases overattention to your own intellectual processes, rather than the bases upon which they have been developed, is a mistake. What you are ideally aspiring toward is an elegantly presented flow of logic, effectively illustrated with sufficient samples from the data to show the genesis and evolution of that logic. In other words, you guide your reader along the trail rather than spending your time making assurances that it exists.

Emden and colleagues remind us of the "moral imperative placed on the researcher that makes honesty and prudence in their publications as significant as the findings themselves" (Emden, Hancock, Schubert, & Darbyshire, 2001, p. 210). When you write well, and have access to a wide range of data bits within which to ground your case, you actually have a range of options for presentation of your findings. If you become overly invested in a particular metaphoric representation or conceptual image, it is often quite possible to dredge up sufficient instances that "might" be representative to write up a case that looks convincing. This is why it is essential to maintain an integrity of purpose in both the doing and the writing of your interpretive description—so that the product of your efforts can be taken up in the manner you intended, entered into the continuing knowledge dialogue within your discipline, and put to some use in solving human problems. If you find that you are "using" the qualitative research enterprise to serve some other purpose, you may have disserved yourself and your profession.

When an interpretive description not only illuminates some aspect of human experience that had been less visible or even obscured previously, the criteria by which the quality of the product will be judged will depend upon the reader's capacity to follow the design choices you made, the manner in which you enacted them, the sample to which you had access, the data you extracted from that sample, and the sense you made of that data. Following the audit trail does not require full knowledge of each of these elements (or qualitative research could never be disseminated in a 15-page manuscript). However, the logical association between each element and all others must be convincingly apparent in the written report. The reader who understands the ingredients of a qualitative product must be able to see evidence that you gathered data in a particular manner, and that you systematically reflected on those data until you were able to articulate a meaningful way of explaining its core elements. You will convey this through your language selection, the way you link ideas together, and the integrity of the explanations. When the reader can see that the product is well -made, the findings arrive at some measure of credibility. Thus, much of your capacity to make visible the logical path you have followed rests with the conceptual structure and narrative form within which your findings are made manifest.

Avoiding Predictable Problems

Complicating the writing process are a host of avoidable problems that are worth mentioning as you strategize your writing process. Depending on the type of written product you are generating (e.g., a brief journal report or a much longer doctoral dissertation), you'll want to familiarize yourself with the form within the genre and the general expectations or requirements that may constrain your options. In most instances, you'll find that you can work within a fairly broad range of constraints. However, a journal style format that insists you articulate the hypothesis being tested may pose a real challenge!

Misuse of Metaphor

Although most interpretive description does not seek overarching metaphoric representation of phenomena as its primary objective, the use of metaphor is undoubtedly an important mechanism for articulating interpretive material. It permits us to explain one thing in terms of another, elucidating elements in relationship in a manner that may be quite difficult to communicate otherwise. However, if metaphor is to be used in the writing, it is essential that it be handled thoughtfully and intelligently (Sandelowski, 1998). Metaphors privilege certain angles of vision and even values about a thing (and in the qualitative health research world, it seems they are more popularly used to make inferences about heroic acts, objects of beauty, or wonders of nature than defeat, decrepitude, or turmoil!) (Thorne & Darbyshire, 2005). The slanted perspective that a metaphor suggests can do injustice to the totality of an inherently complex phenomenon. We might find it morally satisfying to claim that breast cancer is about spiritual growth, for example, but for many women, pain, disruption to normal daily life, and threats of mortality still take precedence. In writing about metaphoric representations in qualitative reports, Sandelowski reminds us that "Metaphors are supposed to make things cohere: to link the parts to a whole" (1998, p. 379). Mixed or aborted metaphors therefore detract from coherent rendering. An overstretched metaphor becomes absurd, while one that is underemployed becomes relatively meaning-less. When the "balancing act" becomes an "obstacle course," we lose our capacity to "harvest the wisdom" it was intended to nurture!

Descriptive or Analytic Excess

Lofland and Lofland (1995) point out that both description and analysis (interpretation) in excess can detract from the quality of a qualitative research report. Qualitative researchers often cite Clifford Geertz (1973) to justify the inherent value of "thick description," even when their reports actually reflect large quantities of the more "thin" variety rather than descriptions that meet strong interpretive criteria (Denzin, 1989; Sandelowski, 2004a). As Wolcott has commented, this all too often takes the form of "heaped data" (1994, p. 13), from which the reader is expected to draw his or her own conclusions.

The opposite problem is also the case in some qualitative reports, where analytic procedures are themselves reported as findings. Where there is too little description to support the interpretation, the treatment of data can become the primary focus of a research report. Write-ups structured around lists of processes, themes, categories, or dimensions without showing what connections there might be between them or how they might contribute to some larger whole will not have met their objective, and may reflect the author's conviction that his or her thinking, and not the phenomenon at hand, is at the center of the inquiry (Sandelowski & Barroso, 2002).

Conceptual Confusion

To this point, we have not addressed the issue of bringing ideas from the literature into the written report of findings. This too is a matter of preference, with some scholars choosing to generate findings prior to discussing them on the basis of the available literature, and others choosing to integrate the two operations. For the purposes of this book, I have chosen to separate them into distinct chapters, so as to address different kinds of issues arising with each. Because generating a written report of findings and critically interpreting its central claims in the light of extant knowledge are two quite different intellectual operations, I tend to encourage newer researchers to keep them separate until they know how their own thinking patterns will be influenced by the attempt to combine them. In most instances, even when a final written report reflects a blend of the two, one mental operation has preceded the other.

Where literature is brought into the presentation of findings, however, it is of utmost importance that you avoid slippage and drift with your conceptual representations. Whether your write-up has been organized around a conceptual description or a thematic summary, you will have used conceptual language in your interpretive synthesis of findings. Once having done this, you must remember that you have chosen words and phrases to denote ideas, and it is the ideas that remain the important element of the finding. Because you quite likely selected terms that distinguished what you were doing from "common" language within the field, the terminological variation is not in and of itself a finding. Instead, you have an obligation to pay serious attention to the points that other authors have been trying to make in using their particular terms, and not read any particular importance into the apparent similarity or difference. If you have capitalized on a conceptual term to reflect a core element of your findings synthesis, then you no longer have license to use that same term as it would be used in common parlance. In other words, having designated a central authority to a term, you can't change your mind and have it mean something different.

Although this is not by any means an exhaustive list of the hazards to avoid, thinking about these issues should orient you to the purpose that is driving your study, your options for conveying to your eventual reader the passion and enthusiasm you have for your topic, and the technical strategies with which you can optimize the successful report of findings. Although one can say a lot about how and how not to write, in the end it is the attitude and application of the writer that creates the written work. Remember that it takes patience, practice, and persistence. Writing qualitative findings is quite a different form of writing than any other. It takes a serious investment of yourself, engagement of your conceptual mind, and the ability to step outside your embedded perspective to appreciate the manner in which your writing will be received in the wider world. Mentors, guides, and editorial critics may well add valuable support along the way, but it is ultimately you driving the logic and determining how best to convey in written form what it is that you have discovered.

In the preceding set of chapters, we have focused our attention on the doing of interpretive description. Now, as we head into the final chapters of this book, we shift our angle of analysis into the larger issues of what it is that the interpretive description means within the larger knowledge context.

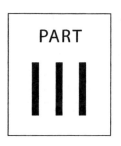

PART

III

INTERPRETIVE DESCRIPTION
IN CONTEXT

Making Sense of Findings

Although completing the written report of your findings tends to feel like closing the curtain on a five-act play (complete with an expectation of joyous applause), there is more to be done before the interpretive description is complete. As with all research, the findings from your study require thoughtful examination, reflection, and reinterpretation within the context of what else is known about the phenomenon before you can legitimately report what it is that the study "means" in the larger scheme of things. In this chapter, we'll consider the processes of working with your findings: "discussing" them in the context of other literature, drawing conclusions on the basis of them, and considering what (if any) implications might derive from what you can conclude. Each of these requires an understanding of the nature of the knowledge world into which you hope your findings will effect an entry. The extent to which that is achievable will depend in no small measure on your capacity to step back and appreciate the limits of your findings within that wider context.

Discussing Findings

Once your findings are neatly displayed in written form, they have taken a shape and structure that permits you to focus your attention on what kind of contribution they might make to advancing knowledge. Having had to draw your findings report to a close, you will have found yourself forced to summarize what the key points of your write-up were, and what the central conclusions to your account contained. You will have had to explicitly distinguish that which has been "found" from that which has merely been observed. From there, you now need to make some decisions about which of those elements that have been found deserve further examination in the context of what's known.

Identifying What's Important

Although everything in your written report is undoubtedly important to you, and an indispensable element of the whole—lived, embedded, embodied subjective human experiences that you have been faithfully recording—some of the ideas will be objectively more "important" than others. Determining which ideas constitute the appropriate level of importance for further discussion requires that you understand the nature of your research question, the knowledge community from which the question arose, the construction of your data, and also the interpretive processes through which you transformed them into findings.

You may find, for example, that certain of your findings take on importance because they depart in some manner (subtly or dramatically) from what the literature or your clinical impressions might have led you to expect. If this is the case, before determining whether the findings are or are not important, you might need to ask yourself about the extent to which this departure might reflect your sampling limits or the passage of time since the original observations were made and results published. In other words, simply noticing the unexpected does not necessarily make a finding important, since there may be self-evident reasons why your findings and those of others are different. However, where there is no apparent explanation, variance from the expected can lend importance to certain elements within your findings, including those that may not have been represented as prominent within your conceptual conclusion.

The central theme or conceptualization that represents your findings will usually be an important component of what deserves discussion. Certainly you will want to examine what it means that you synthesized component parts in a particular manner while others observing similar parts may have made different choices. However, if your conceptualization reflects an abstraction or a metaphoric representation, then it is the idea that is being represented that deserves this further attention. For example, if you conceptualized the coming-of-age experiences you have been studying as being "like a butterfly," it may not be important that others have referenced the metamorphosis as relating to a moth or to a flower blossoming, but rather what will be relevant is the key properties, qualities, or elements that the interpreter was trying to emphasize in articulating those analogies. As you will find when you go back to the literature with fresh eyes, what authors sometimes claim to be their main finding is more properly understood as the platter upon which they presented it, the serving dish upon which they were able to display that which made it what it was. You'll want to ensure that you don't make that error, and so discussion time becomes the opportunity to reflect differently on your findings and understand them in another way. To some extent, this explains why it is quite difficult to discuss findings at the same time as you are generating the initial written report of them, and why most scholars create an explicit separation between the two intellectual processes.

Getting below the signifiers and into the meaning becomes an important part of determining what truly is important and worth further discussion within your study. You might ask yourself:

- What are the main messages here?

- What is it that I know now, having done this study, that I did not know before?

- Or, that I did not know in the same way?

Thus findings can sometimes be distilled into "take home messages" that represent the essence of the ideas that you have so carefully documented in meticulous detail. While it can be disconcerting to think that you have expended so much effort and come away with essentially a "sound bite," it can be useful to remind yourself that if you cannot sum up the point of a paper in a single sentence, you may not yet know what the point of that paper was (Sandelowski, 1994a, p. 376).

Considering your own findings in this light, you will identify a handful (my term for roughly two to five major themes) within your study that deserve further attention and consideration in light of the wider knowledge universe. You will need to understand the basis on which you have decided to address them in this way, and make that explicit to your reader. In this way, you are setting the stage for the conversation you and your theoretical reader are now entering.

Deciding How to Interpret

When you bring your findings onto the ballroom for their debut performance and invite them to engage with other dancers, you will want to choose quite carefully with whom you wish them to interact. Certainly you have a ready troupe of performers already gathered for the purposes of the literature review with which you began your study; however, you are also likely to want to seek out new players, the exciting and exotic experts whose relevance has emerged during your absence, or whose relevance has come into focus because of your immersion in rehearsal. Recognizing that you are looking for different kinds of literature

---

TEXT BOX 11.1

The Transition into Cohabitation with Family

Firbank and Johnson-Lafleur used interpretive description to learn more about the nature of the transition when an elderly person and his or her family caregiver decide to move into a shared residence. Interviewing both elders and family caregivers, these authors found this transition to be characterized by a staged process of moves in and out of cohabitation until eventually the situation stabilized. Periods of crisis were interspersed with phases of relative calm, and decisions regarding relocation often took shape over a lengthy period of time. Within the population Firbank and Johnson-Lafleur studied, which included families of both French-Canadian and Haitian origin, the availability of home care services did not seem to play a major part in shaping relocation decisions. For most families, there was a strong preference for consensual decision making, and when relocation was decided, it was generally justified by health concerns, a belief in reciprocity, and family tradition. Despite the uncertainty of the transitional time, it did seem to prepare both elders and families for the emotional and practical challenges of living together.

Firbank, O. E., & Johnson-Lafleur, J. (2007). Older persons relocating with a family caregiver: Processes, stages, and motives. *Journal of Applied Gerontology, 26*(2), 182–207.

---

for different elements of the discussion of findings is an important component in thinking through the potential scope and breadth of interpretation available to you.

Original Literature The "old friends"—those key pieces of empirical knowledge that you will have critiqued and challenged in justifying your study in the first place—have likely been with you, at least in the background, throughout your research process. In fact, recognizing where your observations may have been similar to or different from what they reported may have played a role in shaping what you conceptualized as findings. In general, we do not "find" what we are told exists and predictably observe; rather, we "find" the unexpected, the interpretively distinct, and the deeper linkages, those elements beyond what would have been self-evident or commonly understood. This might explain, for example, why those researchers in a particular era found growth and spiritual transformation among women with breast cancer—not because the threats to femininity and longevity were no longer present, but because they were so strongly anticipated. Remembering this, it is important to be able to dig deep into (and beneath) the minutiae of the findings that have been reported by others at the same time as we take an objective and distant view of their conclusions.

Thinking about the original literature that you reviewed in this manner, you will be able to see options well beyond the unfortunate and formulaic ritual of reporting whether your findings did or did not "fit" the findings of others. While that observation about degree of fit in general is worth making, it is unlikely of any real interest to your reader whether your findings support, or are supported by, the findings of others. Rather, in the kind of empirical work that interpretive description entails, you are attempting to reintroduce yourself to those sources for the purpose of deepening "meaning."

When you return to the original literature, your motivation is to see whether there is anything within your new findings that sheds a different angle of vision on what you thought you understood from them in the first place. You may find it useful to reflect on individual pieces of literature one at a time, but also to consider the "weight" of the literature as it would have oriented you toward various emphases, directions, or perspectives. If you are reporting on aspects of your findings that are distinct from what was previously reported, you'll need to reflect on whether that distinctiveness is relevant. For example, if you strategically selected your sample on the basis of guidance provided by previous researchers on the important limits of their own, then it may not be of importance that you saw something that they didn't. Essentially, you and they are in agreement as to what improves the angle of vision, not in disagreement as to what was found.

New Literature   Ideally, your immersion in the process of your interpretive description will have brought you to some insights, observations, and ideas that were not entirely anticipated on the basis of your review of the original literature. Indeed, if all there was to find was what one might have expected, then one could question your justification for doing the study in the first place. So beyond reconsideration of the insights within the original literature on the basis of new angles, nuances, or discoveries that your research process has uncovered, you are likely to want to extend your interpretation of findings into bodies of literature that might not have seemed so centrally important in the first place.

For those who have constrained their academic involvement within a specific disciplinary context, it can be daunting to have to consider reading outside the discipline. Fortunately for those in the health professions and in other applied disciplines, interdisciplinarity tends to be as fundamental as breathing, and the idea of "borrowing" knowledge from a wide range of disciplines is not foreign or frightening. However, the idea of interdisciplinarity and the enactment of a thoughtful interdisciplinary interpretation can be two quite different things.

None of us can ever be equally expert in all knowledge traditions; nor can we fully embody the ideational structures of all disciplinary perspectives. What we can do, however, is strive toward a reading knowledge of central ideas within other disciplines as they pertain to the substantive issues with which we are concerned. So, for example, where an applied social anthropologist is studying the cognitive processes involved in workers adapting to a new organizational structure, he or she might well draw upon psychological theorizing as well as applied knowledge in the field of organizational behavior management. If, however, his or her discoveries had to do with changed identities resulting from these experiences, he might also find important insights in such fields as nursing or social work, where considerable attention has been paid to the impact of altered life circumstances upon identity. Thus, the capacity to imagine where other scholars might be doing work that has relevant parallels and from which alternative insights may derive is an important element in what makes a good piece of interpretive description truly excellent. While focused, disciplinary knowledge is a useful commodity, the capacity to look into its inevitable blind spots comes from having braved the wider world of general ideas. The best of researchers are those who also read, listen, and engage in that wider world.

There are many ways in which you can expand your capacity to consider new and potentially relevant bodies of literature, and developing the habit of capitalizing on them is a useful adjunct to your research effectiveness. Much research takes place in and around a university context, and universities are hotbeds of ideas and inspiration. By sharing your general ideas and emerging findings with others, and explicitly soliciting their ideas about other forms of inquiry or bodies of knowledge you may not yet have tapped, you can signal your enthusiasm to your wider community and increase the likelihood that colleagues will share suggestions, no matter how wild and wonderful they might seem. Although many of us in the initial phases of our research are hoping not to find any more new literature, in these concluding phases the motivation is quite the reverse, and putting out feelers may well yield interesting results. When you present preliminary findings, such as to a graduate seminar or a group of professional colleagues, don't miss the opportunity to ask for ideas as to

- What else might this mean?
- What other fields of study might be coming up with ideas that have some parallels?
- What else do my findings make you wonder about?

Although the prospect of developing a full reading knowledge of other disciplines keeps many researchers from peeking out from their usual reading comfort zone, there are many efficient techniques for getting an initial "feel" for what might be there. Given a hint of a possible link between your findings and the knowledge that is developing within a certain discipline, it is often possible to locate among your academic, collegial, or even social networks someone who knows something about the area and can give you some starting direction. What seems self-evident to those in one discipline is often quite foreign to another, so calling up the civil engineer who lives down the block may help you find language or reference points about a concept such as "tension" from which you can locate current thinking about particular problems that may inform the human experiential analogy. Also, don't underestimate the potential importance of that which may be core or basic knowledge within another discipline. If you have uncovered important new insights about the way in which people facing childbirth or terminal illness reference transcendental meanings within their experience, you may find it helpful to understand how anthropology has dealt with the role of myth within culture, or the insights that comparative theology offers with regard to human variation in matters of the spirit. Sometimes, an exploration that begins with those "101" core texts within the discipline can orient you to the language, the key thinkers, and the branches of study whose insights may help broaden your discussion beyond the base from which you began.

Another aspect of knowledge that may have had short shrift in your original literature review and that you may wish to bring forward in the discussion is the body of quantitatively derived knowledge that has been developed in the field. While you may find the idea of measurement antithetical to the grounded, holistic conceptualization you are concerned with, what it is that people have found to measure and what they think they have learned on the basis of that measurement is an aspect that deserves careful consideration. As we'll consider further in the final chapter when we discuss evidence, much of what we need to know in order to advance the applied practice fields depends upon skilful integration of understandings that are only possible on the basis of the distinct methodological traditions. Those who study individual cases cannot presume to claims about larger populations, while those who refine the art of measurement cannot help us understand the unique and particular. Many of the really important questions actually require both species of knowledge. By bringing into the discussion the current wisdom from the other side of the scholarly community, you begin to see a wider potential for interpretive description results.

The new literature that you invite into your discussion of findings offers a real advantage in allowing you to interrogate what you have learned from diverse perspectives and to imagine what might be possible if alternative research agendas were followed in the future. A thorough and thoughtful discussion of this type will often make explicit the possible advantages of following several distinct lines of inquiry as the field of knowledge develops. In enlisting this new literature to assist with discussion of your findings, it is important to recognize that it was there all along and it was you who hadn't quite noticed. This recognition becomes important in that it shapes the manner in which you reference new ideas—not as support for your findings, but rather as additional angles of vision from which to reflect on the potential meaning and impact of the ideas that you have added. Your discussion then might broaden to a consideration of the potential contribution that bringing the two bodies of literature together might make, or to the future potential of a reframed research agenda. While this exploration in new literature may not yield perfect matches, it does tend to help you move in your thinking beyond repetition of your current study and into a more robust program of research.

Extending Interpretation In considering the challenge of interpreting your findings, it is useful to reflect for a moment on the larger context of what the term "interpretation" has come to signify within the scientific and philosophical worlds in recent years. Beyond the "interpretive slant" that is inherent in the very idea that knowledge from the perspective of those involved is a worthy objective, there is an "interpretive turn" that reflects an explicit and volitional application of specific ways of handling ideas when we make sense of that human subjective material. In some scholarly communities, interpretive approaches have become explicitly associated with a postmodernist perspective that may be quite distinct from what you think you are doing with your interpretive description research. Shusterman aligns current trends in interpretive theorizing with loss of faith in foundationalism, realism, and objectivity. He notes,

> Having abandoned the ideal of reaching a naked, rock-bottom, unmediated God's-eye-view of reality, we seem impelled to embrace the opposite position—that we see everything through an interpretive veil or from an interpretive angle. (1991, p. 103)

TEXT BOX 11.2

Becoming Caregiver

O'Connor used interpretive description to examine the ways in which family members of elderly individuals come to be identified as the family caregiver, with all of the associated roles and responsibilities. Through her interviews with these individuals, she found that they did not make a conscious decision to assume that role but rather had it placed upon them gradually by situational factors and the expectations of others. Many found the idea of caregiving to be quite different from their previous role identification as family member, and for many the implications of being a caregiver became apparent over time. Although most had not sought the role, it did bring practical benefits in assuming control over some decisions. At the same time, it was typically fraught with tensions and contradictions, and adopting the caregiver identity precluded the option of giving one's own needs priority. A subtle benefit of the caregiving role, however, was that it provided an alternative form of relating when prior ways of familial relating were no longer possible. By allowing them an objectivity about their loved one's situation, it helped them cope with the situation. O'Connor's findings permit a heightened understanding of the implications of this important identity transition in the care context.

O'Connor, D.L. (2007). Self-identifying as a caregiver: Exploring the positioning process. *Journal of Aging Studies, 21*, 165–174.

This form of interpretation reminds us of the hermeneutic circle in which we come to understand something in a particular way because of who we are, not because, necessarily, of any inherent or immutable properties it possesses.

As was explained in Chapter 1, the world of ideas within which the interpretive description methodological approach was developed pertains to application rather than the primary objective of theorizing. The world of application draws inspiration and often useful insight from its dance with the theoretical world, but at the same time refrains from fully committing to the relationship because the everyday practical problems toward which it is directed demand that at least one foot be firmly placed on the solid grounding that there is a "real world" to be dealt with. Because it is a human world, the nature of that real world may be intricately connected with our capacity to know and understand it, but our particular understanding is not the main fascination. Whether certain angles of vision will or will not assist with problem solving keeps us firmly grounded within what we consider to reflect reality.

In this context, the "interpretive" world becomes a place where we can temporarily assume a standpoint and reflect on "what if" we saw things from different angles of vision. By taking on feminism, post-structuralism, or post-colonialism, for example, as the standpoint from which to examine our findings, we may well find that we can expose new questions or sharpen our focus on certain elements. However, these explicitly "interpretive" stances we might play with do not become our *raison d'être*, but rather serve as yet another lens through which our kaleidoscope of perspective may be enriched.

One way of thinking about the role that interpretation plays with our interpretive description is to consider an important distinction between interpretation and explanation. While we use the two terms colloquially in a similar manner, it is instructive to distinguish explanation as the understanding of causal antecedents and interpretation as delineating the context that may help us understand why something occurred (Roth, 1991). While explanation creates the means of prediction in relation to something like human behavior, interpretation simply helps us better understand the "reasons and rules" surrounding it. The interpretivist world, therefore, "looks for culturally-derived and historically situated interpretations of the social life-world" (Crotty, 1998, p. 67). Debates abound within the literature as to the attitude surrounding how culture and human experience interact. For example, according to Crotty, symbolic interactionism considers culture as the matrix that shapes our lives, while phenomenology recognizes it as giving entrée to a comprehensive set of meanings while simultaneously blinding us to "an abundant font of untapped significance" (p. 71).

Located as a research approach in which the social, structural, cultural, and historical context of human experience is recognized as powerfully influential upon what we know, experience, and think (Garrick, 1999), interpretive description seeks to understand how that context plays out in individual experience to the extent that it can be known. While it uses human experience as its starting point, it is not constrained from considering other dimensions within which that experience may be situated. Thus, it seems necessary and relevant to include within the full interpretation of findings those "explanations" and interpretations that may shed light on what influences are shaping the circumstances and how they may be interacting with one another to mould the manner in which people live and interpret their living. Thus, the bodies of literature within which these interpretive angles of vision

---

TEXT BOX 11.3

The Power of Numbers

Thorne and colleagues used interpretive description to analyze a large data set of interviews with patients about their cancer care communication to ascertain patterns and themes in the reports associated with numerical information. They found that, because patients almost universally experienced cancer as a potential threat of mortality, they were especially vulnerable to acute distress around statistical information. They tended to have significant difficulty making constructive sense of information in numeric form and found themselves calculating and reframing the odds on the basis of a generally limited understanding of probability. Thorne and colleagues found that patients believed that health care providers used numeric information not only to inform their patients but also to manipulate their decision making and manage what they perceived as unrealistic hope. The findings of this study illuminate the precarious balance between hope and despair, and illustrate how powerful a role numerical information pertaining to population-based data can play in shaping the cancer experience of individuals.

Thorne, S., Hislop, G. T., Kuo, M., & Armstrong, E.-A. (2006). Hope and probability: Patient perspectives of the meaning of numerical information in cancer communication. *Qualitative Health Research, 16*(3), 318–336.

---

are developed and explored may well be a useful additional source of inspiration for interpreting findings. At very least, they keep us alert to the context within which our evolving knowledge must reside.

Drawing Conclusions

Although there will have been concluding elements to the final para-graphs of your findings write-up, these are somewhat different from the ideas that we can fully justify as the "conclusions" of your study. Because interpretive description generally taps human experience in context, with the inherent limitations that implies, it is essential that you engage in a distinct process of reasoning before you can generate the "so what" of what you have been studying.

The simple way of saying this is that conclusions are a product of study findings interpreted in the context of the available literature. What that means, however, is that you have recognized the inherent limits of knowledge derived exclusively from the specific perspectives you have had access to in your study (regardless of how meticulously and exhaustively you may have documented them). Understanding that any one study only and exclusively permits a narrow range of conclusions helps you understand why the broadest form of discussion with the literature provides an advantage.

When your findings have revealed elements that have not been reported elsewhere (and your search has been sufficiently diverse to allow you to claim that honestly), then there is very little you can conclude other than the idea that your observation may warrant further investigation in future studies. Unless you can substantiate your suspicion with other empirical work or clinical opinion literature, for example, your conviction that the phenomenon you observed is more widespread than has been previously recognized has very little credibility as a conclusion at this point. What you can do, however, is articulate your observation using the somewhat vague and imprecise language indicative of a question rather than an answer. On the basis of your findings, you might conclude, for example, that "individuals recovering from hip-replacement surgery may experience a form of existential vulnerability that interferes with their ability to fully engage in exercise therapy." This wording allows you to keep the suspicion in play without denying the possibility that your observation may have been an artifact of your particular study at the place and time it was conducted or of your own particular slant as the interpretive instrument. Your perspective may have been shaped by one or two particularly vivid and compelling accounts that led you to explore more deeply for this kind of phenomenon within your sample. Whether there were some unique aspects to your sample that might account for a difference between it and a more general population remain a matter of pure conjecture. Does the bedside manner of the particular surgeon doing these operations in your city increase the likelihood of post-operative fear? Is the phenomenon you observed one that is common to a wide range of health conditions, just not especially documented in relation to this patient group? So your capacity to read and inquire broadly, to ask questions about what else might be like the phenomenon you observed, or who else might have made observations that resemble what you have documented in some manner will help you put some perspective on whether your research product constitutes a potentially useful clinical observation or a profound, groundbreaking new discovery.

Where your findings can be deeply interpreted in the context of significant bodies of literature, especially where such bodies combine robust

TEXT BOX 11.4

The Impact of Smell and Taste

In this interpretive description, Bernhardson and Tishelman explored patient experiences with the changes in smell and taste that accompany cyclotoxic cancer chemotherapy. Noting that these common changes have been virtually ignored in the literature, the authors sought to learn what they mean in the lives of patients and how these patients manage them over time. They found that, while there was a wide variety in the intensity and sensation of these symptoms, they had a meaningful impact on patients' everyday lives for as long as they endured. They found that smell and taste alterations were not always distinguishable and were difficult for the patients to accurately describe. These authors also documented the profound impact that chemosensory changes had for many patients, inducing a sense of joylessness and irritation, as well as compromising the ability to maintain adequate nutrition. They also reported some of the creative ways in which patients experimented with managing these challenges, including relying on smell and taste memory and modifying their food preparation techniques. The authors concluded that their findings will help legitimize the seriousness of these kinds of symptoms, prompting clinicians to talk about them to their patients and to become interested in seeking solutions.

Bernhardson, B.-M., & Tishelman, C. (2007). Chemosensory changes experienced by patients undergoing cancer chemotherapy: A qualitative interview study. *Journal of Pain and Symptom Management, 34*(4), 403–412.

empirical and theoretical literature, the fruits of your interpretive description may be considerably more amenable to strongly articulated conclusions. What you are stating, in coming to such conclusions, is not what the world knows now as a direct result of your singular study, but what your study, in combination with a body of knowledge, allows us to feel relatively confident about and to understand in a particular way. Confirming that what has already been well established also applies to your particular sample is not in and of itself terribly satisfying, but locating your findings within a larger context does create the platform upon which you can justify the particular extensions, elaborations, and enrichments that your study findings contribute. Generally, the more intricately linked your data elements, and the more coherently articulated the relationships between them, the more likely you are to use literature to your advantage as a basis upon which to articulate credible conclusions. Further, among the more important kinds of conclusions you may have come to is recognition that knowledge relying upon other angles of vision (such as quantification or clinical wisdom) may have some important blind spots and limitations. Your most meaningful conclusions may be those possibilities that you make visible by virtue of the particular approach you have taken to surfacing the kind of knowledge that clinicians sense and human experience confirms.

Finally, in articulating conclusions, it is useful to remind ourselves that interpretive description makes no claim upon "truth," and conclusions deriving from it must always be expressed in a manner consistent with that understanding. Unlike other forms of science, within which "certainty" represents a shared understanding that there are immutable facts, even as imperfect as our capacity to know them may be, interpretive approaches at best produce knowledge claims that are inherently particularistic, relativistic, and evolving according to changing circumstances (Forbes et al., 1999). The conclusions we draw on the basis of our interpretive description research, therefore, must always reflect a respect for the context within which they were derived.

Considering Implications

Implications for Further Research

In keeping with the scientific tradition in which it is embedded, one in which the thirst for knowledge is understood to be infinite, all research ends with a consideration of what the next logical steps might be if we are to advance knowledge in this field even farther, and explicitly what is it that the new study has contributed that may inform future inquiries. Your interpretive description is not complete, therefore, without some mention of what future research might arise on the basis of what you have learned in the course of your study.

In general, the very weakest suggestion you can propose is that someone ought to replicate your study in a larger context or with some different features to the sample. While this may well be your own aspiration, it is very unlikely that replication, in and of itself, justifies further research. Further, recognizing the interpretive tradition within which you have conducted your study, it actually makes little sense to suggest that someone could start where you began and think the same way you did about the phenomenon of interest given new material. Consequently, starting your discussion of implications with a replication recommendation flags to your audience that you may not be thinking deeply about what it is that you have produced or what implications it might really have for further inquiry.

What becomes a more convincing argument in favor of future research is the specific questions you have brought into focus and curiosities you may have inspired through your thoughtful interpretation of your results in the context of the wider body of knowledge. Where your study has revealed a new dimension of a phenomenon, an alternative conceptualization that ties together elements that were previously understood as merely coincidental, another layer of experience that has not yet been fully developed within the clinical knowledge, then you have a powerful basis upon which to make recommendations for further studies. What ought to guide you, however, is the original research problem with which you entered the field: What did you think needed to be known, and who needed to know it? Orienting your future research recommendations around the larger goals of that original clinical question will allow you to articulate the potential role of this study within what could become a much more vigorous, focused, and productive program of research—a challenge that you yourself might take up, or one toward which you might invite your audience.

The most useful recommendations will be those that reflect awareness of the limitations of your study approach and the advantages that other methods or designs might afford. Thus, rather than encouraging your practice community to focus its attention on interpretively oriented inquiry, you will have made a much more important contribution if you can suggest various angles of the overall problem that might strategically be addressed using the full range of inquiry approaches. The point, after all, is meaningful knowledge, and in the world of practice application, that will always and inherently mean population-based generalizable knowledge in tension with individually oriented experiential and interpretive analysis.

In many instances, the data base you will have constructed for the purposes of your research will have angles unexplored and depths untapped as you have focused your attention on the aspect that your research question directed. At the point of completing your study, you have an intense and immersed knowledge of what is there, and what that kind of engaged, interactive data collection approach can yield. Thus, another element of your recommendations for future research may well revolve around related questions that you now believe ought to be asked, either of your data set at a later time or by future studies more specifically directed toward the topic. As many researchers working in the field of qualitative and interpretive inquiry have observed, the rich content inherent in so many data bases would provide an important comparator for later secondary analysis so that the implications of the historical context in which it was created can be illuminated with the informed perspective of time (Mottier, 2005). In proposing such future possibilities, you are doing justice not only to the conclusions you were able to reach, but also to those that you may have realized were beyond your grasp because of the context and conditions of your study.

Implications for Everything Else

In the world of the applied disciplines, it is almost inevitable that a research report will go further than simply recommending future studies, but will also comment on a range of other recommendations that derive from having done the research. Because the practice mandate is the "so what" of the applied world, reporting back to your community what you think ought to be done differently in such domains as education, practice, service delivery, or even policy seems essential. It is important to remember that, for the nonapplied disciplines, making recommendations for action on the basis of a single study would be heresy. And this attitude of humility will serve you well in addressing the matter of implications if you keep the inherent limits of your interpretive description study firmly in mind.

That said, you will likely believe that there are some aspects of your study that those in your profession really ought to understand so that their practice can be more sensitive, better informed, or increasingly thoughtful. You may even feel that the insights you have uncovered are of such importance that they ought to be taught to new practitioners or embedded within the policy frameworks where their work will be conducted. While your enthusiasm may be commendable, try to avoid the temptation to use your study as a platform from which to argue all of the opinions and preferences you have developed in the course of your professional career as a vision for a better world. Although those passions have their place and deserve expression in the appropriate venue, suggesting that they have now been rendered "evidence based" by virtue of your interpretive description may inflict an injustice upon the credibility of the qualitative inquiry genre.

Disseminating Knowledge

While the written report, in the form of a publishable paper or volume, is the standard form of communicating what has been learned from a qualitative project such as an interpretive description study, you might consider a number of alternative approaches for sharing the insights you have gleaned with relevant audiences. Because the challenge of knowledge transfer is well recognized within the scholarly and policy communities, it seems important to reflect on how the research you have conducted on behalf of an applied discipline might actually find its way back into the world of practice knowledge. In this chapter, we'll briefly comment on some of the standard and innovative mechanisms that have been used by various applied qualitative researchers to address this problem, hopefully inspiring you to generate your own ideas for ways of getting your newfound knowledge into the hands of those who stand to benefit.

Professional and Scholarly Communications

Most researchers will find the professional and scholarly communities the most obvious first point of communication. Giving some thought to when, how, and why you want to interact with these audiences will help you make effective decisions about what to do with your research findings.

While there is no "right answer" for how to take your findings into the wider domain of knowledge dissemination, it is well worth reviewing some options. The ones that will be best for you will often depend on where you are in your career, what your career aspirations are, and what role your study is playing in the development of that career. While those issues should never be the sole driver of dissemination activities, they do become important considerations. What might be appropriate early in your academic career—when you want to show the capacity to bring a project through to publication for the purpose of establishing your research track record or obtaining tenure—might not be the best option later on when you are concerned with building a comprehensive research program or mentoring junior scholars. Further, these issues shift over time, between disciplines, and in response to a wide range of contextual factors such as the economic drivers for research. It is always wise when setting out in your career to find thoughtful mentors with whom you can have frank conversations about the implications of various choices as you develop your career foundations. Practicalities aside, I would hope that what generally drives your decisions is a conviction about

- which are the really important fields of study,
- which questions within them demand urgent attention, and
- how best you might use the privilege of being able to conduct research to make a significant difference where it counts.

Publication Options

Sadly, while some interpretive description projects could become fascinating books, and the extended space afforded by the book format does permit the development of a truly in-depth exploration within the research report, the world of publishing today is unlikely to make the book format the preferable choice for most applied researchers. Although they do represent a marvelous tradition within the social and health sciences (Wilson & Hutchinson, 1997), monographs reflecting a single study are likely to be those that are developed on the basis of larger projects, with extensive sampling, and on topics that are of general public interest. In this case, writing them up "as research" may not serve the marketing needs of the publisher, and so the fact that the findings derive from a rigorous empirical investigation may have to be relegated to the appended material. In general, you would consider a book when the topic is of great popular interest, when you can anticipate a ready market, and when you are not terribly concerned about the opinion of an academic audience. Although there may yet be disciplinary variation in this regard, the applied health field seems increasingly indifferent to the book format as a way of communicating research results.

Journal articles have become the mainstay of research publication in recent times. The number of professional and scholarly journals has proliferated rapidly, and the range of available publication venues means that you are likely to have multiple options. Journals differ in terms of their scholarliness, their intended audience, or their prestige value. An important distinction is whether or not they are "refereed," which refers to the established convention of acceptance based on the recommendations arising from blind peer review. Most academic institutions consider refereed papers to be inherently stronger, in that they have attained publication on the basis of a process that is well understood (leaving aside the recent critique that has been made with regard to how rigorous and meaningful the peer review process may have become!) (Hojat, Gonnella, & Caelleigh, 2003).

At one time, an important consideration in selecting a journal was its intended audience. You decided on the professional group you most wanted to speak to and published in the journal that group was most likely to read, regardless of its prestige value. In our rapidly changing information age, however, the critical factor tends to be in which referencing systems it is indexed. While some indexes are discipline-specific, those most valuable for publishing purposes may be the more general ones, which will often be the point of first access for those seeking out literature on your topic.

Impact factor is a consideration of particular concern to those pursuing research or academic careers in which their scholarly productivity will influence their career progress. This reflects a numeric measure of the frequency with which the journal articles are accessed and cited. While this too is a rather contested issue (there are various ways in which journal impact factors can be artificially inflated by such things as editorial policies), it generally helps others distinguish those journals that are widely read from those that are local, obscure, or not yet well established. A related issue to consider in selecting a journal is its acceptance rate. While it can be daunting to submit a manuscript to a journal with a low acceptance rate, the quality of the papers accepted is likely to be higher, and this will be well recognized within your disciplinary circles. So although publishing your research report in the *North Overshoe Winter Chronicles* may be an efficient way to get it into press, it is not going to speak to your audience in the same manner as would a paper in *Science* or the *New England Journal of Medicine*. Since what you are aiming for is likely somewhere in the middle of these polar extremes, you'll want to weigh all of these factors in your consideration.

All journals have author information readily available, most typically on websites or in the journal itself. Pay careful attention to author guidelines for such issues as length, format, and writing style. If the word limit constraints are too narrow for you to do justice to your study, search for a journal whose guidelines are more compatible with the products of qualitative inquiry.

In writing up your research, use what you have learned as an informed reader to guide your sensibility about how much depth and detail you can permit yourself within the confines of the journal article format. Although you will never be able to say it all, the piece must say enough to convey the logic and significance of the study in order for it to be meaningful. Many interpretive description studies will be amenable to more than one publication, so if you can't reasonably address all that must be said in a single paper, consider how you might divide up some of the ideas or emphases into distinct but linked written reports. It is never appropriate to "salami slice" your study by writing up multiple similar reports with only minor differences, and in no case can any portion of a paper duplicate that which has been submitted elsewhere. Duplicate publication and self-plagiarism are serious problems. You would not want your reputation to be tainted by the perception that your distinct products were not original scholarship, and you would never want to put yourself afoul of copyright law. Thus, consider publishing more than a single paper where there are distinct elements or angles to be reported, where a secondary analysis has been conducted on the same data set as a result of the findings from the primary study, or where there is a methodological or clinical application that becomes a meaningful companion to the more formal research report. In all instances, acknowledge the other papers that relate to the same study with formal citations, and inform the journal editors where there is any potential overlap to determine how best to reference it.

When writing up your interpretive description report for publication, it is important to acknowledge methodological direction and how you enacted it in your design. Because interpretive description is a logic model rather than a cookbook, you cannot simply reference a source and assume the reader understands what choices you have made and why. In many instances, you will also have drawn upon techniques or processes from beyond interpretive description per se. In such instances, to avoid peer reviewer misunderstanding, I have found it helpful to explicitly name and reference interpretive description as the methodological approach, and to note that this tradition is consistent with design options that are "informed by" certain other traditions.

Presentation Formats

Scholarly and professional presentations are another primary mechanism for disseminating research findings. Numerous conferences invite submission of abstracts and provide opportunities for those accepted to present their work in oral or poster format. While some conferences and meetings attract disciplinary audiences working across a full range of topics, others are specific to an interdisciplinary audience within a substantive field. Some are targeted toward researchers, and others attract a mix of clinical/professional and academic folk. It is useful to consider who it is you wish to be speaking to when you make decisions about which conferences you will submit to, and how many conferences you can reasonably manage. They tend to be expensive, time-consuming, and busy events (often with most participants vying for attention with their own presentations), and so ensuring you attend the right ones is wise.

The oral presentation is the standard mechanism for most scholarly communities—this despite the weight of evidence that suggests it is among the least effective ways to communicate information. In modern conferences, you will be given strict time limits, and it is prudent to plan carefully so that you can adhere to them. Going overtime and being hauled off the podium does not lend credibility to your work, and ensuring that you leave time for questions and discussion if at all possible is the best way to create audience engagement with your work.

Some people are excellent extemporaneous speakers, and can work with slides or minimal notes. Others (especially newer researchers) may do better with a prepared (and timed) speech; however, if you do, try to ensure that you do not revert to pure reading, and practice working from your text in a manner that is lively, accessible, and amenable to engaging with the audience. Audiovisual materials, including PowerPoint slides, can be a marvelous visual adjunct to oral presentations. Alternatively, they can be frustrating, mindlessly tedious, or distracting. Make use of the many available resources to ensure that you align your audiovisuals with the rest of your presentation, use each element wisely, and understand how to judge the impact of your presentation package on your audience. Knowing your particular skills and limitations will help you prepare a successful oral presentation.

Poster presentations are another attractive mechanism for sharing your findings. In general, they afford a more generous timeframe in which to engage with your audience, and allow for more one-to-one networking with those who self-identify as being interested in your field of study. You'll maximize these advantages if your poster looks professional, uses images as well as text to attract attention, and contains sufficient information to explain your work without going overboard with detail (Wilson & Hutchinson, 1997). Many poster sessions allow you to share more detailed written reports with interested conference participants, or hand out your business card for continuing connections.

Another dissemination mechanism to consider is the symposium—a presentation option available in a number of conference contexts. A symposium tends to be a collection of paper presentations on a particular theme, developed as a coherent package, and structured so as to maximize interaction between presenters and with the audience. While being invited to participate in a symposium in your field can be an excellent way to engage actively with other researchers, designing your own forum and inviting those scholars you'd most like to involve in it is also an option. Despite all of our many ways of creating connection, face-to-face human dialogue still creates an important basis for truly productive ongoing professional connections.

Knowledge Transfer Projects

Increasingly, research funding bodies and policy makers have been strategizing new mechanisms to bring the ideas deriving from research into the relevant practice communities. Thus, beyond presenting your findings to other researchers, you may want to seek out involvement in various knowledge transfer projects as opportunities become available or to generate your own such initiatives. Such projects may support active involvement of practice professionals within ongoing programs of research, multi-site teams of scholars, and clinicians working together to solve system-level problems, or the development of blended clinical research units within which the needs of the practice community explicitly drive and support the activities of the researchers. Because it has not always been easy for members of the research community to find optimal ways to package their findings that are relevant and meaningful to the practice sector, or to appreciate the compelling barriers to the application of research findings, these kinds of initiatives may reflect a powerful emerging way to bridge the two worlds. From the perspective of interpretive description research, active ongoing engagement in this kind of activity provides a tremendous advantage in exposing you to the experiential reality of those "inside" and to informing your ongoing interpretive understanding of the larger social, historical, and cultural context within which practice occurs. This level of engagement enhances the angle of vision with which you can identify and work with relevant research questions.

Public Domain Communications

Although many researchers never consider dissemination options beyond the standard "presentation and publication" venues, it is becoming increasingly important that research and the world it presumes to
serve are in close interaction with one another. Thus many qualitative
researchers have explored alternative forms of disseminating research
findings as a way to inform, educate, and invite a wider community
into the dialogue.

Artistic Renderings

Across the health and social sciences, there is a relatively recent trend
involving representation of qualitative study findings in various artistic
formats, including the novel, poetry, dance, painting, sculpture, documentary drama, and theatrical performance. To some extent, these approaches reflect an enthusiasm for modes of representation that depart
from those of traditional science, where it was thought to misrepresent
human experience and, in some instances, reproduce social inequities
(Sandelowski & Barroso, 2002). In addition, they have been considered
essential to the goal of reaching audiences beyond those who access
a scientific format (Schwandt, 1994) and for communicating those aspects of new knowledge that are difficult to convey linguistically or best
experienced in expressive form (Norris, 1997). In a certain manner of
thinking, science and art reflect a kinship in their mutual search for
realities that represent forms of truth (Thorne, 1997). As Sandelowski
argues, "Artistic truths are often more true to life than scientific ones,
providing us with visions of human nature more resonant with our
own experiences than any psychological, sociological, or other conven-
tionally scientific rendering of it" (1994a, p.127).

A significant problem with artistic renderings, however, is that one
faces a considerable challenge knowing precisely what one is to do
with them (Schwalbe, 1995). As a society, we know how to judge the
credibility of a scientific product, and we have an entirely different set
of assumptions and standards for how the worth of an artistic product
ought to be determined. When something straddles that line, the evaluative criteria become much more slippery, such that what might be
good theater could well be misguided interpretation of findings, and so
on. As Norris points out, artistic forms thrive on creating heightened
ambiguity, and thereby invite the kind of misreading that might be of

considerable concern (Norris, 1997). Thus, although there is considerable appeal to the idea of experimenting with alternative representations of some of our research findings, such enterprises are not to be undertaken without caution and a healthy respect for the rules of engagement with which we entered the scientific endeavor in the first place. The host of epistemological and ethical issues raised by these alternative modes give cause for significant concern, especially in the context of the practice professions, where such findings were intended to inform our practice.

Despite these challenges, I am aware of some spectacular instances of qualitative research findings dissemination in the artistic mode for which there is evidence that the intended message can be handled responsibly (Thorne, 2000b). The first is a play based on the phenomenological research of Dr. Vangie Bergum (1997). Set in a hospital delivery room, *A Child in Mind* captures the experience of being transformed from woman to mother by juxtaposing the experiences of six very different women as they make that transition. The individual stories reflect the complexities and contradictions of social disparities as well as challenges brought about by such factors as new reproductive technologies. Highlighting issues of social justice and self-exploration, the play stimulates thoughtful deliberation and, as part of the production, the audience is invited to participate in a discussion that includes both researcher/authors and actors. Another is a theatrical production based on the work of Dr. Ross Gray and colleagues (Gray, et al., 1998) based on qualitative research into complexities inherent in living with metastatic breast cancer. Entitled *Handle with Care*, this production was developed in a series of workshops involving the research team, an artistic director, and a group of actors who themselves had metastatic breast disease. Drawing on segments of raw data as the basis for thematic excerpts, the team scripted a play in two formats, one intended for health care professionals and the other for community audiences. It has been performed widely, and the systematic analysis of evaluative feedback data following each production has allowed the team to understand the impact that it has had on distinct audiences (Gray, et al., 2000).

Interpretive description attempts to make visible the commonalities inherent in such complex phenomena as the intricate dynamics of human relationships and the psychological twists and turns that characterize human experience. It also seeks to reveal their variations as different people experience similar situations in different ways. Thus, doing justice to the findings of an excellent study within the confines of a 15-page manuscript may be impossible. The appeal to explore dissemination methods that afford more depth and more accessibility to all concerned seems a particularly high priority (Morse, 2000; Sandelowski, 1998).

Engaging the Media

The trick to engaging the media, whether it be newspaper, radio, television, or other formats, is developing the art of reducing your research to a slogan or sound bite and communicating about it in a manner that is both true to the essence of the work and accessible and interesting to a wide audience. While there may be occasions when the media find you, more often it will be you who must do the hard work to build relationships and confidence (May, 1997). Many universities and institutions have public relations departments that are of infinite assistance in helping you learn how to attract media attention, package your ideas in a manner that they can manage, and conduct yourself in an interview situation. Seek out these resources and take full advantage of them, as working with the media requires a range of competencies, infinite diplomacy, and a dose of hardnosed persistence.

An important element of media work is timing. While you might want wide exposure for the study you intend to conduct for the purpose of recruiting volunteer participants, your intentions are unlikely to represent the kind of story that would attract media attention. Instead, try to find the angle of your study that will be of general interest, work to reduce it to manageable messages, and find a legitimate way to convey it with a sense of urgency. When you help the media understand your story, assist them to make a report interesting by providing them with real people to interview and factual background information to substantiate your claims, you increase the likelihood of your work being picked up and reported. If possible, also try to align reporting with an event that can engage the reading or listening audience—a public lecture, a new development in service delivery, or an active public policy consultation.

It is also worth mentioning that there are always risks associated with media engagement. You typically have limited (if any) control over what is done with your material, and once it is in the public domain, it can be widely transmitted without your knowledge or consent. While you can ask to see prepublication drafts or to confirm quotes, these privileges are rarely guaranteed. Your best strategy, therefore, is to be carefully prepared, to provide as much useful information as the situation requires, and to try to ensure that nothing you say or communicate would get you in trouble if taken out of context. Beyond that, it may be wise to develop a thick skin and a good sense of humor.

Making Use of Information Technology

Many research projects and programs are now finding websites a marvelous way to disseminate study findings. While the internet is increasingly a site of virtual participant observation and research engagement all on its own, it has tremendous advantages for controlling the information that is disseminated, showcasing varying levels and layers of information depending on self-selected interest, and creating a communication network around your study findings.

On a website, you can engage your audience in getting to know the researcher (or the research team), in understanding the motivation underlying a program of research, and in following the progress of the program over time. While it is typically not appropriate to publish tentative findings in this manner, there is often a considerable amount of information that can be formatted to meet the needs of the professional community and the general public. Over time, as the prevalence of open source journals increases and the accessible information proliferates, you'll have expanded options for linkage with other resources, networks and services through the website mechanism. Thus, your study report can also become part of the larger project of serving the practice communities and the clients of their services that inspired your original research.

A word about copyright. As you publish from your studies, do consult with journals to learn how and under what circumstances electronic formats become publicly available. Some journals have a time period after which you can share these materials fairly freely, and increasingly some are making open access available from the outset. These are changing times, and the knowledge dissemination process will be changing with them.

Community Engagement

Not to be ignored are the full range of other options that you may have available if you stretch your creativity and think about where people affected by the issues you are concerned with may reside or congregate. In many communities, there will be various groups of the general public always interested in learning something new from the research community. Assuming your work is in an area of human interest (and almost anything that taps human subjective experience as a source of primary knowledge has potential!), you may well find that local libraries, community centers, faith communities, or service clubs are eager for a volunteer speaker or guest at their meetings. These kinds of community engagements can be invaluable in mobilizing word-of-mouth communication, profiling your work, and even garnering support for your future research. The scholarly generosity they imply shapes the context for future researchers as communities increasingly recognize that the research community has a human face and is working with a range of approaches to solve important problems. There may also be community groups for whom your particular topic is a primary focus of concern. Patient support groups or consumer advocacy groups would be examples of places where reaching out and developing relationships could be of special significance.

In my own work, I have found that speaking to both specific and general community groups often proves multifaceted in its impact. Members of the audience are often surprised that some of the human elements of experience with health and illness are of concern to the professional community, and feel energized to hear results that validate subjectivity as a relevant source of insight for health service. Further, I have found such audiences to be an endless source of informal credibility checking, as audience members share with me their own similar or contrasting experiences.

CHAPTER THIRTEEN

Enhancing Credibility

Although a concern for credibility has been embedded throughout the previous chapters in relation to each element of the research process, here we reflect upon qualitative research credibility in the larger context of applied disciplinary knowledge. Interpretive description seeks access to an important kind of knowledge about human subjective experience. However, we must remember that its products are not inevitably accurate, relevant, or even necessarily socially responsible, and the knowledge deriving from them will be no more or less credible than knowledge derived from a range of alternative sources. Thus, it is essential that we have access to thoughtfully developed quality criteria to assist with both reading this kind of research and guiding the conduct of it (Engel & Kuzel, 1992; Kuzel & Engel, 2001; Morse, Barrett, Mayan, Olson, & Spiers, 2002; Popay, Rogers, & Williams, 1998; Seale & Silverman, 1997).

Interpretive description was specifically designed to address what had been identified as an epistemological confusion within the qualitative health research field that appeared in the form of weak or ambiguous methodology resulting from an incomplete shift from a quantitative to a qualitative philosophical orientation (Burns, 1989; Leininger, 1994). This was particularly the case in the context of inappropriate application of quantitative quality measures to what ought to have been recognized as an entirely distinct epistemological enterprise.

The ideas contained in this chapter draw heavily on a previously published examination of options for understanding and judging quality within the constraints of the qualitative traditions, and how we might distinguish mediocrity from excellence (Thorne, 1997)[1]. In that earlier writing, I tried to synthesize accepted approaches to qualitative credibility to show how various scholars had tried to translate the

[1]Permission to reprint substantial parts of the original has been provided by Sage Publications, Inc.

imperative of the quantitative "holy trinity" of reliability, validity, and generalizability (Kvale, 1995) into a more compatible philosophical orientation. I used that synthesis as a basis from which to consider the difficulties associated with articulating a methodological "gold standard" within qualitative research in general, and tried to extract some guiding principles that could be developed into a mechanism for comprehensive critique of the quality of qualitative research products. It was my hope in that work, and remains my hope today, that we can find ways to articulate the intricate blend of artistry and the science that interpretive description represents, and thereby render that distinctive perspective increasingly meaningful within the evidentiary context of our practice disciplines. As Elliott and Williams have so eloquently expressed it, "The ultimate paradox is that qualitative inquiry is impossible—both conceptually and practically—yet it still goes on. It must do so if the professions . . . are to advance" (2001, p. 181).

Quality Considerations

Leininger's classic attempts to distinguish critique from evaluation (Leininger, 1968; Leininger, 1994) position critique as the product of a review by someone of recognized authority rather than a matter of comparison against some general evaluative standard. This view assumes the value of applying the critic's "areas of expertise, intellectual astuteness, and philosophical commitments" to the quality judgment (Leininger, 1994, p. 98). However, assuming the imperative that we find mechanisms beyond the stature of an individual critic to decide upon the quality of a work, a more salient approach to credibility assessment would include elements of conventional evaluation to detect evidence of theoretical strength and extend upon that with some form of critique such that the nuances and qualities beyond mere competence also find purchase within our quality considerations. From this angle, critique of qualitative research blends knowledge of the evaluative criteria of qualitative research with a solid foundation in the disciplinary domain for which the knowledge is claimed, combined with the skill set of critical judgment (Berkwits, 1998). Just as the sommelier commands an intimate knowledge of the technology and the artistry of winemaking in order to appreciate subtle distinctions that would escape an ordinary wine drinker, an expert critique of qualitative research demands broad knowledge of the substantive field in which the research attempts to gain acceptance (Parse, Coyne & Smith, 1985).

Despite the emphasis on the stature rather than the ideas of the critic, Leininger's perspective effectively orients us to a kind of evaluation that extends beyond adherence to a set of external standards for methodology and toward a more grounded appreciation for the nature of the knowledge toward which the methods are applied. The importance of extending traditional evaluation into the domain of a more subtle critique can be illustrated with reference to qualitative inquiry within the health sciences. The researcher who presents qualitative research findings to a health science discipline understands that the state of knowledge development is such that research results may well find their way into clinical applications regardless of the researcher's explicit assumptions about their origins. Thus, the standards for health science research must be quite different from standards, for instance, in literary criticism. Health science disciplines exist because of a social mandate that entails a moral obligation toward benefiting individuals and the collective. This factor inherently alters a health science researcher's disciplinary responsibility in such a way that it extends beyond the reach of traditional evaluative criteria and into the domain of how findings might reasonably be interpreted or even used. Thus, an appreciation for the credibility of qualitative research within the health sciences properly extends beyond mere consideration of adherence to the methodological rules and toward examination of the much more complex question of what meaning can be made of the research findings (Angen, 2000; Emden & Sandelowski, 1998, 1999).

Evaluation Criteria

While each qualitative methodological tradition includes distinct guidelines by which it may be judged as theoretically, epistemologically, and technically sound, various qualitative theorists have synthesized sets of general principles that are more or less accepted across the qualitative research spectrum. It is to these general principles that we turn when we consider the kinds of evaluative criteria that are typically applied to the products of interpretive description.

Epistemological Integrity

First, all qualitative research is expected to demonstrate *epistemological integrity* in the sense that there is a defensible line of reasoning from the assumptions made about the nature of knowledge through to the methodological rules by which decisions about the research process are explained. For the findings to be credible, the research process must reveal a research question that is consistent with the stated epistemological standpoint and an interpretation of data sources and interpretive strategies that follows logically from that question. We are necessarily suspicious of research in which the findings produce knowledge incompatible with the assumptions implicit in the design, or knowledge that the researcher was predisposed by prior location or bias to uncover. It is therefore essential that qualitative researchers demonstrate an appreciation of the nature of their epistemological positions and create decisional strategies that respect those positions (Koch, 1995; Simmons, 1995).

Representative Credibility

Second, qualitative studies ought to show *representative credibility* such that the theoretical claims they purport to make are consistent with the manner in which the phenomenon under study was sampled. For example, in a phenomenological single-case study of an illness experience, we would not expect claims about shared elements within experience. Similarly, where a grounded study of a phenomenon reflects the basic social processes of a dominant cultural group, we would not accept inferences that the processes are universal across cultures. We therefore recognize that classic conditions such as Glaser and Strauss's maximal variation (Glaser & Strauss, 1966) are required before certain kinds of knowledge claims can be attempted on the basis of qualitative findings. Study findings based on prolonged engagement with the phenomenon are more likely to be afforded credibility than are those derived from more superficial involvement (Erlandson, et al., 1993). To confirm our inherently constructed perception of an event or process, we generally value some form of triangulation of data sources. Similarly, to convey substantive completeness, we expect that qualitative researchers recognize knowledge beyond a single angle of vision, as depicted in the crystal images evoked by advocates of methodological triangulation (Breitmayer, Ayres, & Knafl, 1993; Richardson, 1994; Sandelowski, 1995a).

Analytic Logic

Third, we expect reports of all qualitative studies to reflect an *analytic logic* that makes explicit the reasoning of the researcher from the inevitable forestructure (Miles & Huberman, 1994) through to the interpretations and knowledge claims made on the basis of what was learned in the research. It is never sufficient for a researcher to assure the reader that an inductive reasoning process occurred; rather, we require that evidence of that logic be apparent throughout the report to the degree that we can confirm or reject its credibility (Morse, 1994b). While it is well recognized that there is an inherently emergent nature to good qualitative research (Sandelowski, Davis & Harris, 1989), the adequacy of the decision making process must be accessible to the qualitative research consumer (Burns, 1989). A commonly applied principle is the generation of an audit trail, an explicit reasoning pathway along which another researcher could presumably follow (Erlandson, et al., 1993; Leininger, 1994). Further, the traditional ethnographic principle associated with the value of thick description charges us with crafting reports that ground our interpretive claims in verbatim accounts from our data.

Interpretive Authority

A fourth requirement is that qualitative studies reveal an *interpretive authority*. While we recognize that all knowledge is perspectival, we need assurance that a researcher's interpretations are trustworthy, that they fairly illustrate or reveal some truth external to his or her own bias or experience. For example, while we value a metaphor that makes our understanding of a complex phenomenon coherent, we demand sufficient information about the data in which the metaphor is grounded to be certain that they are not force fitted into such structure (Janesick, 1994). In our evaluation of qualitative studies, we need to be confident as to which claims represent individual subjective truths and which might represent more common truths. Whatever our theoretical views on the question of generalizability, we must be able to grasp the researcher's intentions in revealing knowledge about the particular. Thus, our reports must account for the reactivity that will occur within the research processes (Paterson, 1994). We build in systems to check our interpretations against those of our research subjects (Hutchinson & Wilson, 1992; Schwandt, 1996). We aim toward convincing our audience of our version of truth through what Altheide and Johnson refer to as "validity-as-reflexive-accounting" (Altheide & Johnson, 1994).

The principles we generate to ensure rigor and credibility within our qualitative research processes all derive from an appreciation of the knowledge claims within which a method is grounded and an awareness of the social context into which our research reports will be directed. Taken together, these four principles form the basis for articulating evaluation standards in interpretive description.

Beyond Evaluation

Because we have access to an increasingly sophisticated set of evaluative standards against which research in the various qualitative traditions can be judged, one might be tempted to assume that merely following the guidelines will produce a product of high quality. However, as has been pointed out by several critics, rigid adherence to textbook approaches in qualitative research (i.e., fetishizing method, methodolatry, criteriology) can propagate weakness rather than strength in our research enterprises (Eakin, 2003; Janesick, 1994; Sandelowski, 1993a; Schwandt, 1996). Here, we are entering the world of a more subtle critique of the products of qualitative research, taking into consideration the larger disciplinary, social, and historical contexts within which they were produced.

Moral Defensibility

Qualitative research within the applied practice disciplines aims toward knowledge that would eventually influence one or another form of practice (Simmons, 1995). For example, we seek to understand how people experience certain assaults of the body, mind, and spirit not in and of themselves but because we hope to be able to alleviate unnecessary suffering or harm and promote as much well-being as is possible under the circumstances. Consequently, a criterion against which all health science research ought to be judged is its *moral defensibility*. We need convincing claims about why the knowledge that we are extracting from people is necessary and what will be the purpose in having such knowledge once we obtain it. This principle, which should apply equally within all practice disciplines, extends beyond traditional ethical claims about the protection of our human subjects and into the realm of an appreciation for how knowledge is used in our society (Lipson, 1994). When we do research in sensitive areas (such as communicable diseases, ethnic diversities, or vulnerable populations), we must account for the possible uses of our findings even before we know what they will include (Sieber, 1993). Our rationale must link the findings to a potential benefit for those we serve before we will find it defensible to place any marginalized group at risk of social censure or antipathy because of the new knowledge we extract or because of the manner in which we make the knowledge accessible to those whose purposes may be distinct from a humanitarian health care agenda.

Disciplinary Relevance

As has been emphasized throughout this discussion of interpretive description as an approach to generating knowledge within the applied and practice disciplines, I envision accounting for the ways in which qualitative research findings meet a standard for *disciplinary relevance* as an essential credibility consideration (Thorne, 2001). Beyond the question of whether society requires the knowledge we seek, a critique of our research products properly includes the issue of whether the knowledge is appropriate to the development of the disciplinary science. In Chapter 2, I referred to a case in which a study of career-oriented women with tattoos had found its way into a prestigious nursing journal, provoking considerable negative reaction within the discipline. This case suggested a deeply felt sense that researchers ought to be required to explain the relationship between their research and the disciplinary knowledge they seek to advance before the professions should support otherwise technically competent inquiry.

Pragmatic Obligation

A third perspective from which the credibility of our research can be considered also derives from the special problems inherent in the practical sciences, where matters of truth and opinion often become blurred around the edges. Apart from any knowledge claims within a health science discipline, whether they be expressed as limits to generalizability or a conviction about multiple coexisting realities, an agreement about what seems real and valid is prerequisite to action. This *pragmatic obligation* reflects the inherent tension within practice realities, in which respect for the uniqueness of individuals creates sympathy for an idealist epistemology at the same time that the moral mandate of a practice discipline requires usable general knowledge. Qualitative health researchers cannot therefore put forth their findings with the comfortable assurance no one will apply them in practice before they become scientifically "proven." Rather, recognition of a practice mandate demands a position that no new idea should be understood as purely theoretical and therefore incapable of rendering harm. Thus, researchers in this field are obliged to consider their findings "as if" they might indeed be applied in practice.

TEXT BOX 13.1

Sustaining Hope

Using interpretive description, Davison and Simpson explored the perceptions of patients with end stage renal disease with regard to how what their professional health care providers say and do affect their ability to hope. Knowing that conversations about prognosis and end of life care have become a moral mandate of health care professionals, Davison and Simpson talked to patients about their experiences of these conversations and their relationship to maintaining hope. Finding that hope was highly personal and shaped by the patients' individual values, the authors also discovered how central hope was to their capacity to engage in advanced care planning. They were able to document, from the patient perspective, a number of options for initiating conversations, providing information, and engaging in advanced planning that would enhance rather than diminish hope. These results create the foundation upon which to raise challenges to current disclosure practices and to find alternatives that may be ethically and psychologically more appropriate.

Davison, S. N. & Simpson, C. (2006). Hope and advance care planning in patients with end stage renal disease: Qualitative interview study. *British Medical Journal*, doi:10.1136/bmj.38965.626520.55 (published 21 September 2006).

Contextual Awareness

A fourth domain inherent in an assessment of research credibility is the *contextual awareness* revealed by a qualitative researcher. The epistemological claims within which qualitative research methods are grounded solidly locate the new knowledge within the society that constructs it. Even so, many qualitative researchers seem not to recognize that their own perspectives are inevitably bounded by their historical context as well as by their disciplinary perspective. Developments in the philosophy of science make it clear that we simply cannot see what we cannot yet see. While those elements of our social historical context that are apparent to us can be accessed, bracketed, and interpreted, we must accept the continuing probability that we are as strongly influenced by other yet invisible shared assumptions. Because many of our tacit understandings are social constructions, they are likely to be shared by others in the field and even by those we attempt to study. Therefore, our research always has the potential to recreate them "as if" they were factual (Herzlich & Pierret, 1985). It is,

TEXT BOX 13.2

Coming Together

Byrd and Garwick used interpretive description to better understand how Black men and White women in biracial families formed their family identities over time. Drawing on couple interviews of parents of biracial school-aged children, they depicted the processes of developing shared beliefs about roles, relationships, and values within a racial context as one of "coming together." Explaining how these families sought to understand the turmoil their marital choices had created and transcend their society's Black-White racial history, they described a set of processes for articulating the family's biracial standpoint and explaining race to their children across developmental stages. These findings provide a basis upon which nurses and other health care professionals can be attuned to the complex process of constructing a mixed-race family in America, and the implications that this process may have on family health events.

Byrd, M. M. & Garwick, A. W. (2006). Family identity: Black-white interracial family health experience. *Journal of Family Nursing, 12*(1), 22–37.

therefore, imperative that qualitative researchers articulate their findings as contextual in the recognition that many supposed accepted realities will not easily withstand the test of time.

Probable Truth

Finally, an appreciation for the credibility of our qualitative research products demands a reverence for the ambiguous zone of validity and shared reality known in philosophical circles as *probable truth*. As has been pointed out in numerous thoughtful considerations of what validity and generalizability might mean in qualitative research (Johnson, 1997; Kvale, 1995; Lincoln, 1995), no set of standards against which we measure our procedures and products can fully account for the notions of truth or even representativeness within the real world, or ensure complete confidence that any research findings are indeed entirely valid. In departing from a search for absolute truths, as all but the most rationalistic of researchers must, we accept that there is considerable value in recognition of some kinds of knowledge as probable truth (Johnson, 1996; Kikuchi & Simmons, 1996), or the best that we have available until we are confronted with compelling reasons to abandon it. However, we must also recognize that certain kinds of knowledge claims that appear to meet our very best truth criteria may in the end prove untrue (see Wolcott's account of *The Brad Trilogy* (Wolcott, 1994) for an exhaustive treatment of one such example). As Eisner has pointed out, it can be useful to reconstruct our sense of why we do research as an effort not to seek truths but to create meaning, to construct images from which people's "fallible and tentative views of the world can be altered, rejected, or made more secure" (1981, p. 9).

Thus, we arrive full circle in our search for truth standards at the portals of moral defensibility, disciplinary relevance, and pragmatic obligation. A sound critique of qualitative research beyond the surface level of adherence to a set of evaluative criteria will therefore inevitably reflect deep questioning as to why we select certain questions to ask, how we claim the knowledge gained will further certain kinds of meaning, and what might be the implications of acts based on what we have come to believe through the process of research.

The Standards Imperative

On the basis of the arguments presented here, it seems evident that the production of excellent interpretive description, as with all qualitative research, demands the skilled application of fundamental competencies within technique and reason, art and science. An increasingly sophisticated set of quality standards is evolving to provide guidelines for establishing the ambitious levels of rigor and credibility within our work. Despite their obvious utility, such rules and guidelines cannot ensure the excellence of any specific interpretive description investigation, and it rests with the qualitative research community to continue to strive toward higher and higher standards in determining what constitutes a credible qualitative research product and what deserves a proper place within the scholarly and professional knowledge base.

In this discussion, we have depicted qualitative research excellence in the context of the purposes for which new knowledge is sought, our orientation toward the actual and potential applications of the ideas we produced, and our reverence for the complexities of truth claims within the scientific enterprise. As trends such as postmodern emancipatory thought within our research communities and the deconstruction of the conventional distinctions between art and science blur our collective sensibilities around how we know what we know, a solid

foundation upon which to articulate the credibility of qualitative research products is becoming increasingly indispensable. Despite the
many challenges that articulating defensible quality criteria poses, it
will always be important for us to find ways to articulate, to ourselves
and to our wider communities, how it is that we can distinguish good
from bad qualitative research—that which should be taken seriously in
the context of our disciplinary knowledge development and that which
ought to be left on the shelf to gather dust.

Advancing Evidence with Interpretive Description

The products of interpretive description are not in and of themselves "evidence," and their precise role within the larger "evidence debate" is a somewhat complex matter. However, they represent a particular species of knowledge that can be profoundly relevant in shaping the sensitivities of the practice context, and in expanding consciousness of the larger spheres within which the structures of our societies evolve. In this chapter, we'll conclude the discussion of interpretive description with some comments on the evidence culture that has become so dominant in health care and other public policy circles. Into this discussion we'll insert the role and potential of qualitative research in general and interpretive description in particular for contributing to the community of evidence-informed decision making. We'll outline some of the methods and techniques that are being worked out for elevating the potential of individual studies to contribute to a larger qualitative evidentiary conversation. And I will share something of my personal experiences and observations with the potential interaction between interpretive description and social change. Through this discussion, we'll conclude the book by returning to the passion that brought us into the research approach in the first place—working within practice disciplines to try to expand knowledge that has the potential of making a difference.

Entering the Evidence Debate

In recent years, some qualitative researchers have bemoaned the lack of enthusiasm from within the quantitative research community for granting credit to the products of their inquiries. In many instances these commentaries challenge the utility of the "gold standard" by which scientific evidence claims are judged—the hierarchy of evidence (Mitchell, 1999). Within this hierarchy, the products of qualitative research count as extremely weak contributors, if they are even noticed at all (Gray, 1997). Various authors advocate educating the larger world to appreciate the products that derive from the use of qualitative approaches, convincing the scientific community to afford qualitative work its rightful place as important evidence, and indeed challenging policy decision makers to make full use of the body of qualitative research when making evidence-based decisions (Kearney, 2001).

While one can appreciate the frustration (for we do seem to be speaking entirely different languages on the two sides of the methodological divide), I believe that competing for a fixed position within the evidentiary hierarchy and/or uncritically advocating the uptake of qualitative research products are misguided and ultimately counterproductive. It may be helpful to remind ourselves of the origins of the evidence debate as it pertains to the applied disciplines (Sackett, Richardson, Rosenberg, & Haynes, 1997; Sackett, Rosenberg, Gray, Haynes, & Richardson, 1996), and to rethink why and how such scholarly contributions as interpretive description might most appropriately be considered in the larger scheme of social and policy decision making.

As with many other areas of public policy, health discourse has become powerfully influenced by expectations around evidence-based decision making (Ray & Mayan, 2001). This trend reflects an increasingly pressing public demand for accountability around allocation of precious resources, and also a progressive distrust that public officials and systems will always make decisions in the people's best interests. This emphasis on that which can be established on the basis of evidence grew out of an acknowledgment within the professional health community that even experienced and apparently expert clinicians could be misled by pattern recognition and perpetuate practices that were unsound, ineffective, or, at times, even dangerous. What an individual clinician with the very best of intentions might subjectively understand as true based on clinical judgment developed over an extensive period of time could, under some circumstances, be completely wrong. Continuing the practice of radical mastectomy for noninvasive breast cancer long past the time at which evidence clearly favored less mutilating procedures is one such instance.

Understanding that background, we can appreciate the importance of the evidence-based practice movement's goal of finding mechanisms for accessing shared truths about which we can have the highest degrees of confidence. Thus, this hierarchy of evidence represents an estimation of the distance between the finding and the possibility of human error or methodological artifact. Organizing what is known according to those aspects about which the objective knowledge is quite clear and those about which we can suspect trends or patterns becomes an important device for focusing the conversation (Madjar & Walton, 2001). That does not mean, however, that only double-blinded randomized controlled trials (RCTs) and systematic reviews count as evidence, but, within the evidentiary analysis, they play a particular (and important) role. Where knowledge development is actually amenable to that form of inquiry, the RCT creates a strong basis for the development of an increasingly widespread agreement on certain parameters of the problem. However, few would make the error of assuming the knowledge all such studies have yielded will inherently be relevant across all contexts or conditions (Johnson, 1997).

It seems naïve, then, to assume that only RCT evidence becomes relevant in decision making. Within health care circles and at public policy tables, there is an increasingly sophisticated understanding that clinical trials, and other forms of strong evidence, are based on particular measures, instruments, and problems. They will have answered some questions about the matter at hand and yet will be completely silent on others. For example, researchers might produce incontrovertible evidence that embryonic stems cells can be cultivated to create specialized cells of benefit to the treatment of an infinite range of diseases, but that evidence does not necessarily lead to the conclusion that it is the right thing to do. Matters of ethics, economics, equity, values, and even human subjective experience become part of the larger context within which important decisions are taken.

What, then, is the potential role for interpretive description within the evidence debate? I suggest that, rather than expending valuable energy demanding that qualitative science be "counted," we ought to learn how to direct our research activities toward addressing the specific evidentiary challenges within each of our practice disciplines (Tarlier, 2005). By this I mean explicitly identifying those elements of our practices about which human experiential knowledge amenable to qualitative inquiry is lacking, tackling head-on the aspects about which our disciplines have a comfortable certainty despite gaps within the experiential dimensions, and grounding our research questions squarely within the issues that have the greatest potential for producing timely and relevant knowledge (Carey, 1997; Olson, 2001). For too long, qualitative researchers have tended to consider all matters of human experience of equivalent relevance in the research enterprise, and topics have not infrequently been chosen on the basis of whim, personal curiosity, or convenience. Within the applied disciplines, I would hope that the era of justifying a qualitative study without a strong relevance argument is nearing its end.

From a policy perspective, this approach would mean familiarizing ourselves with the problems that decision makers face—those aspects about which their inherent uncertainties may be productively addressed through rigorous, systematic, and thoughtful interpretive inquiry tapping the experiential perspective of those most affected (Rist, 1994). Upshur (2001) offers an excellent example of this when he describes using two research papers in teaching evidence-based medicine: One is a meta-analysis of studies showing the lack of benefit of antibiotics for acute respiratory illness and the other a qualitative study of the perceptions of physicians who prescribe them for viral sore throats despite that evidence. In this instance, the qualitative study illuminates the experiential and relational aspects of primary care that explain why the practice persists. By directing attention to the context of the clinical encounter in which the evidence becomes relevant, the qualitative study has yielded knowledge that is easily recognized by all concerned as having importance to the broader question of finding strategies to provide better care.

In health care, for too long we have uncritically accepted the assumption that a single well-designed study can produce sufficiently strong "evidence" to provide certain answers. The evidence hierarchy reinforces this impression that only certain studies attain a pinnacle of "truth." In the legal system, we understand the concept of the "weight" of evidence, or the "preponderance" of evidence, a reference to the idea that there is always and necessarily a vast body of material that together makes up what is understood as evidence. We fully recognize that even the "smoking gun" is rarely sufficient to convict, especially if collateral evidence suggests a different perpetrator. In fact, the legal concept of evidence further presupposes that an unequivocal understanding of it will be infrequent (Upshur, 2001). Rather than arguing the relative weight that ought to be inherently placed on any one kind of research, then, we ought to contribute to a community that becomes increasingly sophisticated in appreciating the limits inherent in all evidentiary sources as well as the tremendous value that a rich, diverse, and robust body of evidence can provide in our quest for useable knowledge.

Putting Research Products to Use

As Estabrooks (2001) reminds us, the larger problem facing us in most instances is not that we have insufficient knowledge, but rather that we lack the will or capacity to put the knowledge we have to good use. This rather humbling thought can serve as a challenge to practitioners of interpretive description, not only to orient their studies toward those issues within which they may have the possibility of influence, but also to build research careers that extend beyond the halls of academe and into the practice arena.

Despite the general challenges of research utilization and knowledge transfer, there is much that thoughtfully planned and conducted interpretive description can do to contribute to the practice context (Olson, 2001; Sandelowski, Trimble, Woodard, & Barroso, 2006). In the health field, for example, many studies are designed for the explicit purpose of uncovering more refined understandings of a health problem from the particular standpoint of the patient. If they are effectively grounded in an informed practice reality, then part of the justification for the study ought to be a reasonable estimation that there is a clinical community that wants to know more about this group of patients or that it can be enticed into learning what it did not think it was missing. When an interpretive description is done well, it not only documents what patients tell us, but it digs below the surface of those tellings to uncover elements of the experience that may help us think entirely differently about the difficulties that they encounter in our care contexts. Because a contextual understanding is fundamental to interpretive description, the findings will have excavated those most vexing aspects of the care context, reframed them into something meaningful, and created alternatives for practice. It has not proven helpful to assume that the obligation rests with the clinical community to seek out and apply our research; rather, it is our duty to ensure that our research is conducted in such a manner that its results will be relevant and meaningful, and that we fulfill our dissemination commitment in the manner that is most likely to entice the opinion leaders within our clinical community to "see the light."

A second way in which our findings can be put to use is in contextualizing and complicating the findings that have derived from quantitative studies. In many instances, population-based studies report behavior patterns but offer no mechanism other than conjecture to explain them. Because of this, studies documenting patterns that appear "irrational" create tensions between the research and the practice community or the public at large. As we know, that which can be documented quantitatively has often been stripped of meaningful variables within its natural context. An increasingly sophisticated reading audience, including the general public, is capable of reflecting critically on this and entertaining competing explanations. In this way, strategically directed qualitative research can enlighten the evidence discourse and ensure that the power of numerical evidence is properly harnessed.

A third mechanism, and one that ought not be underestimated, is what Sandelowski has called "symbolic utilization." By this, she is orienting us toward situations within which qualitative research findings can be used as "a persuasive or political tool to legitimate a position or practice" (2004b, p. 1371). Within the context of the applied disciplines, this has particular appeal for those important practices that are not—and are not ever likely to be—amenable to measurement or quantification, and therefore may be at risk in the context of an overly enthusiastic evidence-based agenda. For example, cost cutting through staff reduction is an ongoing concern within health care. Although it is notoriously difficult to draw causal associations between health care communication and patient outcomes, interpretive description of how that human element of the care encounter informs the patient, prevents predictable problems, enhances service delivery, and mobilizes hope may help organizational decision makers to acknowledge the value of attending to such conditions as staff stability.

In analyzing the emphases of studies published over the first 17 years of the journal *Qualitative Health Research*, Jan Morse notes that qualitative research has made significant contributions to our understanding of ways to delineate health, of impediments to health; ways of understanding illness, of experiencing illness, of experiencing caregiving; and contexts of care (Morse, 2007). As the evidence dialogue shifts from evidence-based to evidence-informed, and the matter of what constitutes top-ranked evidence evolves into a more fulsome conversation about such qualities as verifiability, credibility, and probable truth (as in an agreed-upon conviction that this is the best we have for now), the current tensions between qualitative and quantitative research may resolve themselves. We might envision a preferred future when both qualitative and quantitative researchers eagerly read each other's work, and seek out the opportunity for lively dialogue as to the inherent advantage of seeing the world from these multiple and distinct perspectives. The kinds of issues about which we are equally concerned deserve no less.

Directions in Aggregating and Synthesizing

In recognition of the inherent limits of any single qualitative study and the overwhelming need to develop increasingly complex and comprehensive bodies of knowledge, various authors have proposed directions forward in combining, aggregating, and synthesizing what is already

---

TEXT BOX 14.1

The Attitude of Health Care

Using an interpretive description study design, Thorne and colleagues examined perceptions of health care communication from the perspective of patients with four different chronic diseases. They discovered that general courtesy, respect for the individual, and a commitment to engagement in the encounter were fundamental to all of what patients considered helpful communication. However, they also discerned distinct challenges within the health care provider attitudes about each disease that explained what patients perceived as most problematic about their health care encounters. For each disease, there seemed a characteristic patient "type" that these patients perceived as a negative stereotype interfering with their health care relationships and their consequent capacity to manage their self-care. The findings offer encouragement to the clinical community to appreciate the frustrating nature of self-management for chronic disease and to accommodate that understanding into their communication approaches.

Thorne, S., Harris, S., Mahoney, K., Con, A., & McGuiness, L. (2004). The context of health care communication in chronic illness. *Patient Education & Counseling, 54*, 299–306.

---

known and what is yet to be discovered. One approach is the move from single studies to programmatic research (Sandelowski, 1997). In that they are planned, purposeful, and substantively linked, such enterprises are understood to advance the field toward enhanced practice or policy development. In some instances, these programs explicitly combine secondary analysis of existing data sets with new data collection to expand upon aspects of the original work that deserve further elaboration (Thorne, 1994). This aspect can pose a challenge to qualitative researchers who see their work as having an inherently exploratory, emergent nature that would preclude meaningful planning beyond a single project. However, this aspect does create mechanisms whereby a central focus within a discipline can be examined from multiple angles over time, with the integration of findings culminating in coherent new bodies of substantive knowledge.

Among the most resounding calls to action is the recommendation to develop programmatic research that links both qualitative and quantitative approaches. The basic premise of this challenge is that few of the significant problems within our substantive areas are solvable using singular approaches, and the contrasting attributes of qualitative and quantitative inquiries can become a check and balance for one another as knowledge grows (Bottorff, 1997). Some authors advocate a form of simultaneous methodological triangulation, in which both qualitative and quantitative methods are combined within a single study (Breitmayer et al., 1993; Morse, 1991), while others have critically analyzed the complex issues associated with trying to enact research from fundamentally distinct angles of vision (Sandelowski, 1995c). In response to such challenges, techniques have been proposed for sequential triangulation, in which the results deriving from one approach serve as the foundation for a subsequent phase using a different methodological tradition (Bottorff, 1997; Morse, 1991). Such strategies build in an inherent linkage between distinct sets of findings, and can play a role in the synthesis of knowledge. As methodological work toward this end evolves, there is an increasingly fascinating dialogue on the epistemological challenge of aligning essentially disparate forms of understanding into mixed methods studies. Johnson and Onwuegbuzie (2004) claim "pragmatism as the philosophical partner" of such approaches, acknowledging that while there are not yet perfect solutions, there are highly promising opportunities.

The rapid proliferation of bodies of qualitatively derived findings within health sciences and the practice disciplines over the last generation has led a number of scholars to consider how best to synthesize the accumulated findings from them. Unlike meta-analysis of quantitative studies, in which there are at least some mechanisms for determining like measures, it has proven quite difficult to work out how best to "sum up" diverse products such as those that derive from the various qualitative research traditions (Sandelowski, Docherty, & Emden, 1997b). As might be anticipated, a pure version of phenomenology looks dramatically different from the product of a grounded theory; they are talking different languages, privileging entirely different aspects of thought and action, and ultimately aiming toward quite different purposes. However, despite the methodological claims with which they identify themselves, a great many qualitative research reports produced within the applied disciplines will have departed significantly from their original methodological foundations, and may in fact look much more like a generic qualitative description or an interpretive description. This distance from the social theoretical underpinnings from which the conventional qualitative methods were derived provides an advantage for interpretive description (and related approaches) when it comes time to figuring out what one can do with a substantial collection of such studies.

While methodological direction for qualitative metasynthesis is well beyond the scope of this book (and has been addressed in some detail elsewhere (Paterson, Thorne, Canam, & Jillings, 2001), it seems important here to note some of the promising directions that are evolving to bring together distinct pieces of qualitative inquiry to build more comprehensive, intricate, and robust conceptualizations of the phenomena that concern us. The field of qualitative metasynthesis (which is also known by a wide range of other labels) is rapidly evolving (Sandelowski & Barroso, 2007; Thorne, Jensen, Kearney, Noblit, & Sandelowski, 2004). Although early efforts tended to address "aggregation" of qualitatively derived reports (Estabrooks, Field, & Morse, 1994) or focused on synthesis of small bodies of similar or linked studies (Jensen & Allen, 1996; Sherwood, 1999), the literature now offers an impressive array of highly sophisticated strategic options for generating new knowledge on the basis of large bodies of qualitative inquiry within a field (Finfgeld, 2003). Some approaches emphasize conceptual reintegration of diverse findings (Noblit & Hare, 1988), while others experiment with more summative approaches to understanding the weight of evidence for particular elements across the full range of studies (Sandelowski & Barroso, 2003b). Some metasynthesis methods focus explicitly on synthesis, while others offer mechanisms for critically analyzing the history and tradition of the ingredients that have made up the bodies of qualitatively derived knowledge we now hold (Paterson et al., 2001). Still others advocate combining both an empirical/analytical and a critical/discursive analytical read within a single metasynthesis approach to counter some of the problems that have arisen in relation to the authenticity concern known as the "crisis of representation" (Sandelowski, 2006). Regardless of the emphasis, the scholarly work in this field is making it increasingly apparent that metasynthesis is a highly complex, demanding, and sophisticated programmatic research strategy, and not simply a way to make findings without having to dirty one's hands with "real data." As the qualitative research community matures in its capacity to distinguish legitimate metasynthesis from other less systematic products of literature review, far fewer small studies claiming metasynthesis as their method will likely find their way into print.

A more recent evolution within the methodological literature involves taking up the challenge of research integration, or the application of synthesis techniques to combine what is known on the basis of diverse methods. Forbes and Griffiths, for example, articulate what they refer to as an "evidence synthesis" approach—a systematic, explicit, and reproducible technique which permits both descriptive and predictive aggregation. They argue that, although the methodological challenges are significant, advances in this area are of critical importance in helping us move beyond the competing camps of relativism and positivism:

> On the one hand, we could have produced a clearly defined episte-mological vacuum, represented by the failure to identify evidence convincing to the positivist. Alternatively, we could have filled the vacuum with constructions of reality . . . with no external verifica-tion or consideration of the extent to which this captured the "real" world (2002, p. 153).

Harden and Thomas (2005) describe a "mixed methods" approach to systematic review that capitalizes on emerging approaches within both conventional quantitative systematic review and qualitative metasynthe-sis to extend beyond "what works" to "why." Their approach involves a constant comparative analysis between descriptive and analytic themes searching for matches, mismatches, and gaps between recommendations and demonstrable effect sizes within a particular field. Recognizing that the forms of research across the spectrum are becoming increasingly di-verse, and that conventional systematic review has focused on narrowing down the focus rather than embracing that diversity, they advocate mov-ing beyond the qualitative and quantitative labels toward a focus on distinct kinds of research questions as drivers of epistemologically distinct forms of knowledge, all of which are relevant for comprehensive understanding. Sandelowski and colleagues take this argument one step further in advo-cating a conceptualization of "comparability work" in research synthesis involving qualitative, quantitative, and mixed methods studies. By focus-ing on comparability work, they "move the backstage interpretive work of systematic review to center stage" (Sandelowski, Voils, & Barroso, 2007, p. 236). In so doing, they focus our attention on the choices and compromis-es that define the systematic review process, making transparent the "hid-den judgments" upon which the results rest (p. 244). The wonderfully rich and creative evolving body of thought in this field suggests great promise for the future, when the passion and enthusiasm that fuel the qualitative inquiry can be harnessed and applied to an integrated and comprehensive way of viewing the world, with all of its complexities intact.

Looking Forward with Optimism

In the course of my nursing career, I have had the privilege of witness-ing some fairly momentous shifts in thinking within my own fields of professional activity. Although I claim no particular part in having brought them about, my experience has profoundly confirmed my conviction that the knowledge one can obtain through research methods such as interpretive description can and should find a place within the larger community of evidence-based decision making.

When I first approached the study of chronic illness, I approached it as a "living with" sort of problem, assuming that I could set aside medical management and health care system involvement as somewhat incidental to the challenge of "living with" and focus my attention entirely on what was happening within the lives of those affected and their families. However, participants in my very first study in 1982 told me in no uncertain terms that their engagement with the health care system, and with the practitioners within it, was highly influential in determining what it was they had to "live with" and, further, that a surprisingly major component of their story had to do with the disjunctures and disruptions associated with obtaining appropriate care—this in a country (Canada) with universal health care!

Digging further into the subterranean depths of that tension, I came to appreciate that, from the perspective of those who lived with chronic illness, the health care system was both structurally and ideologically founded on a set of basic assumptions associated with acute and episodic illness visited upon people assumed to be essentially uninformed about what they needed and why (Thorne, 1993). These included the idea that patients needed to be protected from their poor judgment and that acute, not chronic, illness was the legitimate priority of a health care system. By exposing these underlying value perceptions, the patient angle of vision helped me appreciate the pervasiveness and entrenchment of shared attitudes underlying what a health care system ought to be and how it ought to function. In this way, a conceptual synthesis of patient experiences based on a rigorous qualitative investigation produced a depiction of the way in which the larger society, with its science imperative and cost-constraint mentality, had inadvertently created a health care system that, by and large, failed to serve the pressing needs of the chronically ill, and consequently its ultimate social mandate for population health. That way of seeing things, once obtained, becomes very difficult to shake. Over the years my conviction strengthened as I saw evidence of these same values embedded across a wider range of global systems. Thus, an interpretive understanding, accessed by virtue of deep immersion with a purposive sample of "everyday philosophers" who had extensive subjective experiential knowledge of what it was like to have chronic illness in modern society, was and remains an important—almost paradigmatic—insight.

Clearly, my studies were merely miniscule drops in the bucket of converging conditions required to change the course of world events. However, they certainly opened my eyes to an increasingly insistent conversation brought about in part by the continuing work of many qualitative researchers within nursing and the allied health disciplines in documenting chronic illness experience across contexts and cultures (Thorne & Paterson, 2000). Further, they alerted me to the vital importance of working together in an expanded capacity with the epidemiological community to wrestle with population health data in such a manner that alternative interpretations of trends can be explored. Prior to this time, much of the relevant research and scholarship that might have informed the larger "chronic illness" knowledge base was obscured by the alignment of most researchers within "organ system" communities, such that scholars working in cardiac disease, cancer, kidney disease, rheumatology and internal medicine were not yet understanding the inherent value in linking their analyses. Once human experiential patterns common to these distinct organ system conditions were effectively documented, a dialogic space was made for active consideration of the implications of these shared elements.

As various governments and policy communities came to conceptualize the enormity of the chronic illness problem, and subsequently to take note of how many of the costly, preventable sequelae were being mismanaged, the insight that current health care systems were fundamentally misaligned with the need began to take hold among the organ systems and population health specialists. Alternative approaches such as the Chronic Disease Management model (Wagner, et al., 2001) began to appear in policy circles and became the foundation for system re-engineering initiatives. While that model may still reflect something of the professional orientation to chronic disease care, it goes a long way toward enhancing an appreciation that the health care relationship—the interaction between the person with an illness and the professional health care provider who guards access to services— is the pivotal intersection between chronic disease management and everyday self-care decision making.

At this stage in my career, I have the privilege of being included in policy making discussions and therefore have access to the human and evidentiary bases upon which such processes play out. I am fully aware that no single interpretive description study or research program could have directly influenced meaningful change. However, I remain convinced that the hard work of qualitative health researchers everywhere, in uncovering and validating these important perspectival matters, has built a health care consciousness within which new ways of doing business make sense and can be adopted. Essentially, health care professionals need confidence that what they are doing is what's right for patients and for the general public. These insights about radical reconfiguration of how we think about and work with chronic illness are consistent with that objective.

The lesson in this account is that interpretive description (for my early studies were such, even when they referenced naturalistic inquiry or other approaches as the best available alternative for articulating their orientation) is a powerful means for surfacing some important and otherwise invisible dimensions of human experience, stimulating a kind of awareness that has the potential to inform thinking and guide disciplinary practice. Over the years that I have worked within the chronic illness field, I have witnessed many changes in the ways in which practitioners interact with their patients, and increasingly, these changes are justified on the basis of the confirmatory evidence that has arisen from the rich and exciting products of qualitative inquiry. On its own merits, interpretive description has little likelihood of directly influencing system level changes, yet it provides an important tool for ensuring that the perspective of those most deeply affected is accessible to the confluence of evidence deriving from multiple angles. Within any high impact decision in the health care policy context, the patient perspective is now valued as a strategically important consideration. Because decision makers are often uncertain about how best to access that perception, and representational politics become a major stumbling block within policy processes, I believe that elevating the patient perspective to the policy platform through rigorous empirical processes is among the most important roles that interpretive description can take on. By systematically surfacing those aspects of reality that are played out in human experience, we illuminate their intricate and marvelous patterns, rendering inherent complexities into a coherence that informs.

For those of us fortunate enough to have found an applied discipline whose social purpose inspires and motivates us, contributing to the generation of new disciplinary knowledge is a privilege of profound consequence. Within our applied disciplinary communities, we have now entered into the exhilarating prospect of developing an evidentiary basis upon which to wrestle with complex human phenomena, uncover the intricacies of their contextual and relational components, and forecast the effects of various solutions upon the kinds of problems we collectively face. We confront this challenge armed with an increasingly sophisticated set of inquiry tools designed to guide applied researchers in the generation of meaningful and essentially useful new knowledge in the service of these disciplinary projects. Interpretive description is an invitation toward the audacity of imagining that we might begin to answer some of our most pressing questions about the mysteries of human experience.

REFERENCES

Aamodt, A. M. (1989). Ethnography and epistemology: Generating nursing knowledge. In J. M. Morse (Ed.), *Qualitative nursing research: A contemporary dialogue* (pp. 29–40). Rockville, MD: Aspen.

Adler, P. A., & Adler, P. (1994). Observational techniques. In N. K. Denzin & Y. S. Lincoln (Eds.), *Handbook of qualitative research* (pp. 377–392). Thousand Oaks, CA: Sage.

Altheide, D. L., & Johnson, J. M. (1994). Criteria for assessing validity in qualitative research. In N. K. Denzin & Y. S. Lincoln (Eds.), *Handbook of qualitative research* (pp. 485–499). Thousand Oaks, CA: Sage.

Anderson, J. M. (1981). An interpretive approach to clinical nursing research. *Nursing Papers, 13*(4), 6–11.

Anderson, J. M. (1989). The phenomenological perspective. In J. M. Morse (Ed.), *Qualitative nursing research: A contemporary dialogue* (pp. 15–26). Rockville, MD: Aspen.

Angen, M. J. (2000). Evaluating interpretive inquiry: Reviewing the validity debate and opening the dialogue. *Qualitative Health Research, 10*(3), 378–395.

Armstrong, M. L. (1991). Career-oriented women with tattoos. *Image: The Journal of Nursing Scholarship, 23,* 215–220.

Artinian, B. A. (1988). Qualitative modes of inquiry. *Western Journal of Nursing Research, 10,* 138–149.

Baker, C., Wuest, J., & Stern, P. N. (1992). Method slurring: The phenomenological/ grounded theory example. *Journal of Advanced Nursing, 17,* 1355–1360.

Baker, L. (2006). Ten common pitfalls to avoid when conducting qualitative research. *British Journal of Midwifery, 14*(9), 530–531.

Bartolomé, L. (1994). Beyond the methods fetish: Toward a humanizing pedagogy. *Harvard Educational Review, 64,*173–194.

Benner, P. (Ed.). (1994). *Interpretive phenomenology: Embodiment, caring and ethics in health and illness.* Thousand Oaks, CA: Sage.

Benzies, K. M., Premji, S., Hayden, K. A., & Serrett, K. (2006). State-of-the-evidence reviews: Advantages and challenges of including grey literature. *Worldviews on Evidence-Based Nursing, 3*(2), 55–61.

Berger, P., & Luckman, T. (1966). *The social construction of reality: A treatise in the sociology of knowledge.* Garden City, NY: Doubleday.

Bergum, V. (1997). *A child on her mind: The experience of becoming a mother.* Westport, CT: Bergin & Garvey.

Berkwits, M. (1998). From practice to research: The case for criticism in an age of evidence. *Social Science & Medicine, 47*(10), 1539–1545.

Blumer, H. (1969). *Symbolic interactionism.* Englewood Cliffs, NJ: Prentice-Hall.

Bogdevic, S. P. (1999). Participant observation. In B. F. Crabtree & W. L. Miller (Eds.), *Doing qualitative research* (2nd ed., pp. 47–69). Thousand Oaks, CA: Sage.

Booth, A. (2005). Using research in practice: Sole searching—Wasting our time? *Health Information & Libraries Journal, 22*(1), 70–73.

Bottorff, J. L. (1994). Using videotaped recordings in qualitative research. In J. M. Morse (Ed.), *Critical issues in qualitative research methods* (pp. 244–261). Thousand Oaks, CA: Sage.

Bottorff, J. L. (1997). Linking qualitative and quantitative research: New avenues for programmatic research. In J. M. Morse (Ed.), *Completing a qualitative project: Details and dialogue* (pp. 227–249). Thousand Oaks, CA: Sage.

Boutain, D. M. (1999). Critical language and discourse study: Their transformative relevance for critical nursing inquiry. *Advances in Nursing Science, 21,* 1–8.

Bowers, B. J. (1988). Grounded theory. In B. Sarter (Ed.), *Paths to knowledge: Innovative research methods for nursing* (pp. 33–59). New York: National League for Nursing.

Boychuk Duchscher, J. E., & Morgan, D. (2004). Grounded theory: Reflections on the emergence vs. forcing debate. *Journal of Advanced Nursing, 48*(6), 605–612.

Breitmayer, B. J., Ayres, L., & Knafl, K. A. (1993). Triangulation in qualitative research: Evaluation of completeness and confirmation purposes. *Image: Journal of Nursing Scholarship, 25,* 237–243.

Brown, J. B. (1999). The use of focus groups in clinical research. In B. F. Crabtree & W. L. Miller (Eds.), *Doing qualitative research* (2nd ed., pp. 109–124). Thousand Oaks, CA: Sage.

Buissink-Smith, N., & McIntosh, A. (1999). Interpretive description: Advancing qualitative approaches in tourism and hospitality research. *Tourism Analysis, 4,* 115–119.

Burch, R. (1989). On phenomenology and its practice. *Phenomenology & Pedagogy, 7,* 187–217.

Burns, N. (1989). Standards for qualitative research. *Nursing Science Quarterly, 21*(1), 44–52.

Caelli, K., Ray, L., & Mill, J. (2003). "Clear as mud": Toward greater clarity in generic qualitative research. *International Journal of Qualitative Methods, 2*(2). *Article 1.* Retrieved Jan 7/04 from http://www.ualberta.ca/~iiqm/backissues/pdf/caellietal.pdf.

Carey, M. A. (1994). The group effect in focus groups: Planning, implementing, and interpreting focus group research. In J. M. Morse (Ed.), *Critical issues in qualitative research methods* (pp. 225–241). Thousand Oaks, CA: Sage.

Carey, M. A. (1997). Qualitative research in policy development. In J. M. Morse (Ed.), *Completing a qualitative project: Details and dialogue* (pp. 345–354). Thousand Oaks, CA: Sage.

Carey, M. A., & Swanson, J. (2003). Funding for qualitative research. *Qualitative Health Research, 13*(6), 852–856.

Chenail, R. J. (1992). *A case for clinical qualitative research*. Retrieved 1(4), Retrieved Aug 10/99 from http://www.nova.edu/ssss/QR/QR1-4/clinqual.html.

Chenitz, W. C., & Swanson, J. (1986a). *From practice to grounded theory: Qualitative research in nursing*. Menlo Park, CA: Addison-Wesley.

Chenitz, W. C., & Swanson, J. M. (1986b). Qualitative research using grounded theory. In W. C. Chenitz & J. M. Swanson (Eds.), *From practice to grounded theory: Qualitative research in nursing* (pp. 3–15). Menlo Park, CA: Addison-Wesley.

Cicourel, A. V. (1981). Notes on the integration of micro- and macro-levels of analysis. In K. Knorr-Cetina & A. V. Cicourel (Eds.), *Advances in social theory and methodology: Toward an integration of micro- and macro-sociologies* (pp. 51–80). Boston: Routlege & Kegan Paul.

Cohen, M. Z. (1987). A historical overview of the phenomenological movement. *Image: The Journal of Nursing Scholarship, 19*(1), 31–34.

Colaizzi, P. F. (1978). Psychological research as the phenomenologist sees it. In R. S. Valle & S. King (Eds.), *Existential-phenomenological alternatives for psychology* (pp. 48–71). New York: Oxford University Press.

Connelly, L. M., & Yoder, L. H. (2000). Improving qualitative proposals: Common problem areas. *Clinical Nurse Specialist, 14*(2), 69–74.

Crabtree, B. F., & Miller, W. L. (1999a). Introduction. In B. F. Crabtree & W. L. Miller (Eds.), *Doing Qualitative Research* (2nd ed., pp. xi–xvii). Thousand Oaks, CA: Sage.

Crabtree, B. F., & Miller, W. L. (1999b). Using codes and code manuals. In B. F. Crabtree & W. L. Miller (Eds.), *Doing qualitative research* (2nd ed., pp. 163–177). Thousand Oaks, CA: Sage.

Crotty, M. (1998). *The foundations of social research*. London: Sage.

Denzin, N. K. (1989). *Interpretive interactionism*. Newbury Park, CA: Sage.

Dickson-Swift, V., James, E. L., Kippen, S., & Liamputtong, L. (2006). Blurring boundaries in qualitative health research on sensitive topics. *Qualitative Health Research, 16*(6), 853–871.

Durrenberger, P. E., & Thu, K. M. (1999). Why we're worried about cultural anthropology. *Society for Applied Anthropology Newsletter, 19*(3), 3–5.

Dzurek, L. C. (1989). The necessity for and evolution of multiple paradigms for nursing research: A poststructuralist perspective. *Advances in Nursing Science, 11*(4), 69–77.

Eakin, J. M. (2003). Reframing the evaluation of qualitative health research: Reflections on a review of appraisal guidelines in the health sciences. *Journal of Evaluation in Clinical Practice, 9*(2), 187–194.

Easton, K. L., McComish, J. L., & Greenberg, R. (2000). Avoiding common pitfalls in qualitative data collection and transcription. *Qualitative Health Research, 10*(5), 703–707.

Eisner, E. (1981). On the difference between scientific and artistic approaches to qualitative research. *Educational Researcher, 10*(3), 5–9.

Elliott, M. S., & Williams, D. I. (2001). Paradoxes of qualitative research. *Counselling and Psychotherapy Research, 1*(3), 181–183.

Emden, C., Hancock, H., Schubert, S., & Darbyshire, P. (2001). A web of intrigue: The search for quality in qualitative research. *Nurse Education in Practice, 1,* 204–211.

Emden, C., & Sandelowski, M. (1998). The good, the bad and the relative, part one: Conceptions of goodness in qualitative research. *International Journal of Nursing Practice, 4,* 206–212.

Emden, C., & Sandelowski, M. (1999). The good, the bad and the relative, part two: Goodness and the criterion problem in qualitative research. *International Journal of Nursing Practice, 5,* 2–7.

Engel, J. D., & Kuzel, A. J. (1992). On the idea of what constitutes good qualitative inquiry. *Qualitative Health Research, 2*(4), 504–510.

Erlandson, D. A., Harris, E. L., Skipper, B. L., & Allen, S. D. (1993). *Doing naturalistic inquiry: A guide to methods.* Newbury Park, CA: Sage.

Estabrooks, C. A. (2001). Research utilization and qualitative research. In J. M. Morse, J. M. Swanson & A. J. Kuzel (Eds.), *The nature of qualitative evidence* (pp. 275–298). Thousand Oaks, CA: Sage.

Estabrooks, C. A., Field, P. A., & Morse, J. M. (1994). Aggregating qualitative findings: An approach to theory development. *Qualitative Health Research, 4,* 503–511.

Fals-Borda, O., & Rahman, M. A. (1991). *Action and knowledge: Breaking the monopoly with participatory research.* New York: Apex.

Feldman, M. S. (1995). *Strategies for interpreting qualitative data.* Thousand Oaks, CA: Sage.

Field, P. A. (1989). Doing fieldwork in your own culture. In J. M. Morse (Ed.), *Qualitative nursing research: A contemporary dialogue* (pp. 79–91). Rockville, MD: Aspen.

Field, P. A., & Morse, J. M. (1985). *Nursing research: The application of qualitative approaches.* London: Croom Helm.

Fielding, N. G., & Fielding, J. L. (1986). *Linking data.* Beverly Hills, CA: Sage.

Finfgeld, D. L. (2003). Metasynthesis: The state of the art—so far. *Qualitative Health Research, 13,* 893–904.

Finlay, L. (2002). "Outing" the researcher: The provenance, process, and practice of reflexivity. *Qualitative Health Research, 12*(4), 531–545.

Fontana, A., & Frey, J. H. (1994). Interviewing: The art of science. In N. K. Denzin & Y. S. Lincoln (Eds.), *Handbook of qualitative research* (pp. 361–376). Thousand Oaks: Sage.

Forbes, A., & Griffiths, P. (2002). Methodological strategies for the identification and synthesis of "evidence" to support decision-making in relation to complex healthcare systems and practices. *Nursing Inquiry, 9*(3), 141–155.

Forbes, D. A., King, K. M., Kushner, K. E., Letourneau, N. L., Myrick, A. F., & Profetto-McGrath, J. (1999). Warrantable evidence in nursing science. *Journal of Advanced Nursing, 29*(2), 373–379.

Friere, P. (1970). *Pedagogy of the oppressed.* New York: Seabury Press.

Gadamer, H.-G. (1975/1985). Rhetoric, hermeneutics, and the critique of ideology. In K. Mueller-Vollmer (Ed.), *The hermeneutic reader: Texts of the German tradition from the enlightenment to the present* (pp. 274–292). New York: Continuum.

Gadamer, H.-G. (1989). *Truth and method* (2nd ed.). London: Sheed and Ward.

Garrick, J. (1999). Doubting the philosophical assumptions of interpretive research. *Qualitative Studies in Education, 12*(2), 147–156.

Geertz, C. (1973). Thick description: Toward an interpretive theory of culture. In C. Geertz (Ed.), *The interpretation of cultures: Selected essays* (pp. 37–126). New York: Basic Books.

Germain, C. (1986). Ethnography: The method. In P. L. Munhall & C. J. Oiler (Eds.), *Nursing research: A qualitative perspective* (pp. 147–162). Norwalk, CT: Appleton-Century-Crofts.

Gilchrist, V. L., & Williams, R. L. (1999). Key informant interviews. In B. F. Crabtree & W. L. Miller (Eds.), *Doing qualitative research* (2nd ed., pp. 71–88). Thousand Oaks, CA: Sage.

Giordano, J., O'Reilly, M., Taylor, H., & Dogra, N. (2007). Confidentiality and autonomy: the challenge(s) of offering research participants a choice of disclosing their identity. *Qualitative Health Research, 17*(2), 264–275.

Giorgi, A. (1970). *Psychology as a human science.* New York: Harper & Row.

Giorgi, A. (1985). *Phenomenology and phenomenological research.* Pittsburgh: Duquesne University Press.

Glaser, B. G. (2002). Conceptualization: On theory and theorizing using grounded theory. *International Journal of Qualitative Methods, 5* (2), Retrieved June 20/05 from http://www/ualberta.ca/ ~ ijqm/(2).

Glaser, B. G., & Strauss, A. L. (1966). The purpose and credibility of qualitative research. *Nursing Research, 15*(1), 56–61.

Glaser, B. G., & Strauss, A. L. (1967). *The discovery of grounded theory: Strategies for qualitative research.* Chicago: Aldine.

Goffman, E. (1961). *Asylums: essays on the social situation of mental patients and other inmates.* Garden City, NY: Doubleday.

Goffman, E. (1968). *Stigma: Notes on the management of spoiled identity.* Harmondsworth, UK: Penguin.

Gray, J. A. M. (1997). *Evidence-based healthcare.* New York: Churchill Livingstone.

Gray, R. E., Greenberg, M., Fitch, M., Sawka, C., Hampson, A., Labrecque, M., et al. (1998). Information needs of women with metastatic breast cancer. *Cancer Prevention and Control, 2*(2), 57–62.

Gray, R. E., Sinding, C., Ivonoffski, V., Fitch, M., Hampson, A., & Greenberg, M. (2000). The use of research-based theatre in a project related to metastatic breast cancer. *Health Expectations, 3*, 137–144.

Gubrium, J. (1988). *Analyzing field reality.* Newbury Park, CA: Sage.

Hamilton, D. (1994). Traditions, preferences, and postures in applied qualitative research. In N. K. Denzin & Y. S. Lincoln (Eds.), *Handbook of qualitative research* (pp. 60–69). Thousand Oaks, CA: Sage.

Hammersley, M., & Atkinson, P. (1983). *Ethnography: Principles in practice.* London: Tavistock.

Harden, A., & Thomas, J. (2005). Methodological issues in combining diverse study types in systematic reviews. *International Journal of Social Research Methodology, 8*(3), 257–271.

Heaton, J. (2004). *Reworking qualitative data.* London: Sage.

Heidegger, M. (1982). *The basic problems of phenomenology.* Bloomington, IN: Indiana University Press.

Heller, A. (1986). The sociology of everyday life. In U. Himmelstrand (Ed.), *Sociology: From crisis to science?* (Vol. 2, pp. 150–163). London: Sage.

Herzlich, C., & Pierret, J. (1985). The social construction of the patient: Patients and illnesses in other ages. *Social Science & Medicine, 20*(1), 145–151.

Hinds, P. S., Vogel, R. J., & Clarke-Steffen, L. (1997). The possibilities and pitfalls of doing a secondary analysis of a qualitative data set. *Qualitative Health Research, 7*, 408–424.

Hodder, I. (1994). The interpretation of documents and material culture. In N. K. Denzin & Y. S. Lincoln (Eds.), *Handbook of qualitative research* (pp. 393–402). Thousand Oaks, CA: Sage.

Hojat, M., Gonnella, J. S., & Caelleigh, A. S. (2003). Impartial judgment by the "gatekeepers" of science: Fallibility and accountability in the peer review process. *Advances in Health Sciences Education, 8*, 75–96.

Howard, M. C., & McKim, P. C. (1983). *Contemporary cultural anthropology.* Boston: Little, Brown.

Husserl, E. (1929/1975). *The Paris lectures* (P. Koestenbaum, Trans.). The Hague: Martinus Nijhoff.

Hutchinson, S. (1986). Grounded theory: The method. In P. L. Munhall & C. J. Oiler (Eds.), *Nursing research: A qualitative perspective* (pp. 111–130). Norwalk, CT: Appleton-Century-Crofts.

Hutchinson, S., & Wilson, H. S. (1992). Validity threats in scheduled semistructured research interviews. *Nursing Research, 41*, 117–119.

Hutchinson, S., & Wilson, H. (1994). Research and therapeutic interviews: A poststructuralist perspective. In J. M. Morse (Ed.), *Critical issues in qualitative research methods* (pp. 300–315). Thousand Oaks, CA: Sage.

Janesick, V. (1994). The dance of qualitative research design: Metaphor, methodolatry, and meaning. In N. K. Denzin & Y. S. Lincoln (Eds.), *Handbook of qualitative research* (pp. 209–219). Thousand Oaks, CA: Sage.

Jensen, L. A., & Allen, M. N. (1996). Meta-synthesis of qualitative findings. *Qualitative Health Research, 6*, 553–560.

Johnson, J. (1996). Nursing art and prescriptive truths. In J. F. Kikuchi, H. Simmons & D. Romyn (Eds.), *Truth in nursing inquiry* (pp. 36–50). Thousand Oaks, CA: Sage.

Johnson, J. L. (1997). Generalizability in qualitative research: Excavating the discourse. In J. M. Morse (Ed.), *Completing a qualitative project: Details and dialogue* (pp. 191–208). Thousand Oaks, CA: Sage.

Johnson, J. L., & Ratner, P. A. (1977). The nature of knowledge used in nursing practice. In S. E. Thorne & V. E. Hayes (Eds.), *Nursing praxis: Knowledge and action* (pp. 3–22). Thousand Oaks, CA: Sage.

Johnson, M., Long, T., & White, A. (2001). Arguments for "British pluralism" in qualitative health research. *Journal of Advanced Nursing, 33*(2), 243–249.

Johnson, R. B., & Onwuegbuzie, A. J. (2004). Mixed methods research: A research paradigm whose time has come. *Educational Researcher, 33*(7), 14–26.

Kaplan, D., & Manners, R. A. (1972). Formal analysis. In D. Kaplan & R. A. Manners (Eds.), *Culture theory* (pp. 162–188). Englewood Cliffs, NJ: Prentice-Hall.

Kearney, M. H. (2001). Levels and applications of qualitative research evidence. *Research in Nursing & Health, 24,* 145–153.

Kikuchi, J. F., & Simmons, H. (1996). The whole truth and progress in nursing knowledge development. In J. F. Kikuchi, H. Simmons & D. Romyn (Eds.), *Truth in nursing inquiry* (pp. 5–17). Thousand Oaks, CA: Sage.

Kleinman, A. (1980). *Patients and healers in the context of culture: An exploration of the borderland between anthropology, medicine, and psychiatry.* Berkeley, CA: University of California Press.

Knafl, K. A. (1994). Promoting academic integrity in qualitative research. In J. M. Morse (Ed.), *Critical issues in qualitative research methods* (pp. 357–374). Thousand Oaks, CA: Sage.

Knafl, K. A., & Deatrick, J. A. (2005). Top 10 tips for successful qualitative grantsmanship (editorial). *Research in Nursing & Health, 28,* 441–443.

Koch, T. (1995). Interpretive approaches in nursing research: The influence of Husserl and Heidegger. *Journal of Advanced Nursing, 21,* 827–836.

Krueger, R. (1988). *Focus groups: A practical guide for applied research.* Newbury Park, CA: Sage.

Kuhn, T. S. (1962). *The structure of scientific revolutions.* Chicago: University of Chicago Press.

Kuzel, A. J. (1999). Sampling in qualitative inquiry. In B. F. Crabtree & W. L. Miller (Eds.), *Doing qualitative research* (2nd ed., pp. 33–45). Thousand Oaks, CA: Sage.

Kuzel, A. J., & Engel, J. D. (2001). Some pragmatic thoughts about evaluating qualitative research. In J. M. Morse, J. M. Swanson & A. J. Kuzel (Eds.), *The nature of qualitative evidence* (pp. 114–138). Thousand Oaks, CA: Sage.

Kvale, S. (1995). The social construction of validity. *Qualitative Inquiry, 1,* 19–40.

Leininger, M. (1968). The research critique: Nature, function, and art. *Nursing Research, 13,* 444–449.

Leininger, M. M. (1985). Nature, rationale, and importance of qualitative research methods in nursing. In M. M. Leininger (Ed.), *Qualitative research methods in nursing.* New York: Grune & Stratton.

Leininger, M. M. (1994). Evaluation criteria and critique of qualitative research studies. In J. M. Morse (Ed.), *Critical issues in qualitative research methods* (pp. 95–115). Thousand Oaks, CA: Sage.

Liaschenko, J. (1997). Knowing the patient? In S. E. Thorne & V. E. Hayes (Eds.), *Nursing praxis: Knowledge and action* (pp. 23–38). Thousand Oaks, CA: Sage.

Lincoln, Y. S. (1995). Emerging criteria for quality in qualitative and interpretive research. *Qualitative Inquiry, 3,* 275–289.

Lincoln, Y. S., & Guba, E. G. (1985). *Naturalistic inquiry.* Beverly Hills, CA: Sage.

Lipson, J. G. (1989). The use of self in ethnographic research. In J. M. Morse (Ed.), *Qualitative nursing research: A contemporary dialogue* (pp. 61–75). Rockville, MD: Aspen.

Lipson, J. G. (1994). Ethical issues in ethnography. In J. M. Morse (Ed.), *Critical issues in qualitative research methods* (pp. 333–355). Thousand Oaks, CA: Sage.

Lofland, J., & Lofland, L. H. (1995). *Analyzing social settings: A guide to qualitative observation and analysis* (3rd ed.). Belmont, CA: Wadsworth.

Madjar, I., & Walton, J. A. (2001). What is problematic about evidence? In J. M. Morse, J. M. Swanson & A. J. Kuzel (Eds.), *The nature of qualitative evidence* (pp. 28–45). Thousand Oaks, CA: Sage.

Maxwell, J. A. (1998). Designing a qualitative study. In L. Bickman & D. J. Rog (Eds.), *Handbook of applied social research methods* (pp. 69–100). Thousand Oaks, CA: Sage.

Maxwell, L. R. (1997). Foundational thought in the development of knowledge for social change. In S. E. Thorne & V. E. Hayes (Eds.), *Nursing praxis: Knowledge and action* (pp. 203–218). Thousand Oaks, CA: Sage.

May, K. A. (1989). Interview techniques in qualitative research: Concerns and challenges. In J. M. Morse (Ed.), *Qualitative nursing research: A contemporary dialogue* (pp. 171–182). Rockville, MD: Aspen.

May, K. A. (1994). Abstract knowing: The case for magic in method. In J. M. Morse (Ed.), *Critical issues in qualitative research methods* (pp. 10–21). Thousand Oaks, CA: Sage.

May, K. A. (1997). The politicking of research results: Presenting qualitative findings in the public arena. In J. M. Morse (Ed.), *Completing a qualitative project* (pp. 329–343). Thousand Oaks, CA: Sage.

Mays, N., & Pope, C. (1995). Observational methods in health care settings. *British Medical Journal, 311,* 182–184.

McCaffery, M., & Beebe, A. (1989). *Pain: Clinical manual for nursing practice.* St. Louis: Mosby.

McPherson, G., & Thorne, S. (2006). Exploiting exceptions to enhance interpretive qualitative health research: Insights from a study of cancer communication. *International Journal of Qualitative Methods, 5 (2).* Retrieved Aug 14/06 from http://www.ualberta.ca/ ~ ijqm/backissues/5_2/pdf/mcpherson.pdf.

Mead, G. H. (1934). *Mind, self and society.* Chicago: University of Chicago Press.

Miles, M. B., & Huberman, A. M. (1994). *Qualitative data analysis* (2nd ed.). Thousand Oaks, CA: Sage.

Miller, W. L., & Crabtree, B. F. (1994). Clinical research. In N. K. Denzin & Y. S. Lincoln (Eds.), *Handbook of qualitative research* (pp. 340–352). Thousand Oaks, CA: Sage.

Miller, W. L., & Crabtree, B. F. (1999a). Clinical research: A multimethod typology and qualitative roadmap. In B. F. Crabtree & W. L. Miller (Eds.), *Doing qualitative research* (2nd ed., pp. 3–30). Thousand Oaks, CA: Sage.

Miller, W. L., & Crabtree, B. F. (1999b). Depth interviewing. In B. F. Crabtree & W. L. Miller (Eds.), *Doing qualitative research* (2nd ed., pp. 89–107). Thousand Oaks, CA: Sage.

Miller, W. L., & Crabtree, B. F. (1999c). The dance of interpretation. In B. F. Crabtree & W. L. Miller (Eds.), *Doing qualitative research* (pp. 127–143). Thousand Oaks, CA: Sage.

Mitchell, G. J. (1999). Evidence-based practice: Critique and alternative view. *Nursing Science Quarterly, 12*(1), 30–35.

Morgan, D. (1988). *Focus groups as qualitative research.* Newbury Park, CA: Sage.

Morse, J. M. (1989a). Qualitative nursing research: A free-for-all? In J. M. Morse (Ed.), *Qualitative nursing research: A contemporary dialogue* (pp. 3–10). Rockville, MD: Aspen.

Morse, J. M. (1989b). Strategies for sampling. In J. M. Morse (Ed.), *Qualitative nursing research: A contemporary dialogue* (pp. 117–131). Rockville, MD: Aspen.

Morse, J. M. (1991). Methods of qualitative-quantitative methodological triangulation. *Nursing Research, 40,* 120–123.

Morse, J. M. (1994a). Designing funded qualitative research. In N. K. Denzin & Y. S. Lincoln (Eds.), *Handbook of qualitative research* (pp. 220–235). Thousand Oaks, CA: Sage.

Morse, J. M. (1994b). "Emerging from the data": The cognitive process of analysis in qualitative inquiry. In J. M. Morse (Ed.), *Critical issues in qualitative research methods* (pp. 23–43). Thousand Oaks, CA: Sage.

Morse, J. M. (1994c). Going in "blind." *Qualitative Health Research, 4,* 3–5.

Morse, J. M. (2000). The downside of dissemination (editorial). *Qualitative Health Research, 10,* 291–292.

Morse, J. M. (2005). Ethical issues in institutional research (editorial). *Qualitative Health Research, 15*(4), 435–437.

Morse, J. M. (2007). What is the domain of qualitative health research? *Qualitative Health Research, 17*(6), 715–717.

Morse, J. M., Barrett, M., Mayan, M., Olson, K., & Spiers, J. (2002). Verification strategies for establishing reliability and validity in qualitative research. *International Journal of Qualitative Methods, 1 (2), Article 2.* Retrieved from http://www.ualberta.ca/~ijqm/.

Mottier, V. (2005). The interpretive turn: History, memory, and storage in qualitative research. *Forum Qualitative Sozialforschung / Forum: Qualitative Social Research, 6(2), Art. 33.* Retrieved April 4/07 from: http://www.qualitative-research.net/fqs-texte/2-05/05-2-33-e.htm.

Mulhall, A. (2003). In the field: Notes on observation in qualitative research. *Journal of Advanced Nursing, 41*(3), 306–313.

Muller, J. H. (1999). Narrative approaches to qualitative research in primary care. In B. F. Crabtree & W. L. Miller (Eds.), *Doing qualitative research* (2nd ed., pp. 221–238). Thousand Oaks, CA: Sage.

Munhall, P. L. (1989). Institutional review of qualitative research proposals: A task of no small consequence. In J. M. Morse (Ed.), *Qualitative nursing research: A contemporary dialogue* (pp. 241–253). Rockville, MD: Aspen.

Munhall, P. L., & Oiler, C. J. (1986). *Nursing research: A qualitative perspective.* Norwalk, CT: Appleton-Century-Crofts.

Noblit, G. W., & Hare, R. D. (1988). *Meta-ethnography: Synthesizing qualitative studies.* Newbury Park, CA: Sage.

Norris, J. R. (1997). Meaning through form: Alternative modes of knowledge representation. In J. M. Morse (Ed.), *Completing a qualitative project: Details and dialogue* (pp. 87–115). Thousand Oaks, CA: Sage.

Nunkoosing, K. (2005). The problem with interviews. *Qualitative Health Research, 15*(4), 698–706.

Oiler, C. J. (1986). Phenomenology: The method. In P. L. Munhall & C. J. Oiler (Eds.), *Nursing research: A qualitative perspective* (pp. 69–84). Norwalk, CT: Appleton-Century-Crofts.

Olson, K. (2001). Using qualitative research in clinical practice. In J. M. Morse, J. M. Swanson, & A. J. Kuzel (Eds.), *The nature of qualitative evidence* (pp. 259–273). Thousand Oaks, CA: Sage.

Omery, A. (1988). Ethnography. In B. Sarter (Ed.), *Paths to knowledge: Innovative research methods for nursing* (pp. 17–31). New York: National League for Nursing.

Outhwaite, W. (1975). *Understanding social life: The method called Verstehen.* London: Allen & Unwin.

Parse, R. R., Coyne, A. B., & Smith, M. J. (1985). *Nursing research: Qualitative methods.* Bowie, MD: Brady.

Paterson, B., Thorne, S., Canam, C., & Jillings, C. (2001). *Meta-study of qualitative health research: A practical guide to meta-analysis and meta-synthesis.* Thousand Oaks, CA: Sage.

Paterson, B. L. (1994). A framework to identify reactivity in qualitative research. *Western Journal of Nursing Research, 16,* 301–316.

Paterson, B. L., Gregory, D., & Thorne, S. (1999). A protocol for researcher safety. *Qualitative Health Research, 9*(2), 272–282.

Patton, M. Q. (1980). *Qualitative evaluation methods.* Beverly Hills, CA: Sage.

Patton, M. Q. (1987). *Creative evaluation* (2nd ed.). Newbury Park, CA: Sage.

Patton, M. Q. (2002). *Qualitative research & evaluation methods* (3rd ed.). Thousand Oaks, CA: Sage.

Pelto, P. J. (1970). *Anthropological research: The structure of inquiry.* New York: Harper & Row.

Popay, J., Rogers, A., & Williams, G. (1998). Rationale and standards for the systematic review of qualitative literature in health services research. *Qualitative Health Research, 8*(3), 341–351.

Popper, K. S. (1972). *Objective knowledge: An evolutionary approach.* Oxford: Oxford University Press.

Porter, S., & Ryan, S. (1996). Breaking the boundaries between nursing and sociology: A critical realist ethnography of the theory-practice gap. *Journal of Advanced Nursing, 24,* 413–420.

Priest, H., Roberts, P., & Woods, L. (2002). An overview of three different approaches to the interpretation of qualitative data. Part 1: Theoretical issues. *Nurse Researcher, 10*(1), 30–42.

Punch, M. (1994). Politics and ethics in qualitative research. In N. K. Denzin & Y. S. Lincoln (Eds.), *Handbook of qualitative research* (pp. 83–97). Thousand Oaks, CA: Sage.

Purkis, M. E. (1994). Representations of action: Reorienting field studies in nursing practice. In P. Chinn (Ed.), *Advances in methods of inquiry for nursing* (pp. 13–31). Gaithersburg, MD: Aspen.

Ray, L. D., & Mayan, M. (2001). Who decides what counts as evidence? In J. M. Morse, J. M. Swanson, & A. J. Kuzel (Eds.), *The nature of qualitative evidence* (pp. 50–73). Thousand Oaks, CA: Sage.

Ray, M. A. (1994). The richness of phenomenology: Philosophic, theoretic, and methodologic concerns. In J. M. Morse (Ed.), *Critical issues in qualitative research methods* (pp. 117–133). Thousand Oaks, CA: Sage.

Reason, P. (1996). Reflections on the purposes of human inquiry. *Qualitative Inquiry, 2,* 15–28.

Reason, P., & Torbert, W. R. (2001). Toward a Transformational Science: A further look at the scientific merits of action research. *Concepts and Transformations, 6*(1), 1–37.

Reed, P. G. (1995). A treatise on nursing knowledge development for the 21st century: Beyond postmodernism. *Advances in Nursing Science, 17*(3), 70–84.

Richardson, L. (1994). Writing: A method of inquiry. In N. K. Denzin & Y. S. Lincoln (Eds.), *Handbook of qualitative research* (pp. 516–529). Thousand Oaks, CA: Sage.

Ricoeur, P. (1981a). *Hermeneutics and the human sciences.* Cambridge: Cambridge University Press.

Ricoeur, P. (1981b). The task of hermeneutics (J. B. Thompson, Trans.). In J. B. Thompson (Ed.), *Paul Ricoeur: Hermeneutics and the human sciences* (pp. 43–63). Cambridge: Cambridge University Press.

Rist, R. C. (1994). Influencing the policy process with qualitative research. In N. K. Denzin & Y. S. Lincoln (Eds.), *Handbook of qualitative research* (pp. 545–557). Thousand Oaks, CA: Sage.

Robinson, C. A., & Thorne, S. E. (1988). Dilemmas of ethics and validity in qualitative nursing research. *Canadian Journal of Nursing Research, 20*(1), 65–76.

Roth, P. A. (1991). Interpretation as explanation. In D. R. Hiley, J. F. Bohman & R. Shusterman (Eds.), *The interpretive turn: Philosophy, science, culture* (pp. 179–196). Ithaca, NY: Cornell University Press.

Russell, C. L. (2005). An overview of the integrative research review. *Progress in Transplantation, 15,* 8–13.

Sackett, D. L., Richardson, W. S., Rosenberg, W. M., & Haynes, R. B. (1997). *Evidence-based medicine.* New York: Churchill Livingstone.

Sackett, D. L., Rosenberg, W. M., Gray, J. A. M., Haynes, R. B., & Richardson, W. S. (1996). Evidence-based medicine: What it is and what it isn't. *British Medical Journal, 312*(7023), 71–72.

Sacks, O. (1984). *A leg to stand on.* New York: Summit Books.

Sanday, P. R. (1983). The ethnographic paradigm. In J. V. Maanen (Ed.), *Qualitative Methodology* (pp. 19–36). Beverly Hills, CA: Sage.

Sandelowski, M. (1991). Telling stories: Narrative approaches in qualitative research. *Image: The Journal of Nursing Scholarship, 23,* 161–166.

Sandelowski, M. (1993a). Rigor or rigor mortis: The problem of rigor in qualitative research revisited. *Advances in Nursing Science, 16*(2), 1–8.

Sandelowski, M. (1993b). Theory unmasked: The uses and guises of theory in qualitative research. *Research in Nursing & Health, 16,* 213–218.

Sandelowski, M. (1994a). The proof is in the pottery: Toward a poetic for qualitative inquiry. In J. M. Morse (Ed.), *Critical issues in qualitative research methods* (pp. 46–63). Thousand Oaks, CA: Sage.

Sandelowski, M. (1994b). We are the stories we tell: Narrative knowing in nursing practice. *Journal of Holistic Nursing, 12,* 23–33.

Sandelowski, M. (1995a). On the aesthetics of qualitative research. *Image: Journal of Nursing Scholarship, 3,* 205–209.

Sandelowski, M. (1995b). Sample size in qualitative research. *Research in Nursing & Health, 18,* 179–183.

Sandelowski, M. (1995c). Triangles and crystals: On the geometry of qualitative research. *Research in Nursing & Health, 18,* 569–574.

Sandelowski, M. (1996). Truth/storytelling in nursing inquiry. In J. F. Kikuchi, H. Simmons & D. Romyn (Eds.), *Truth in nursing inquiry* (pp. 111–124). Thousand Oaks, CA: Sage.

Sandelowski, M. (1997). Programmatic qualitative research: Or, appreciating the importance of gas station pumps. In J. M. Morse (Ed.), *Completing a qualitative project: Discussion and details* (pp. 211–225). Thousand Oaks, CA: Sage.

Sandelowski, M. (1998). Writing a good read: Strategies for re-presenting qualitative data. *Research in Nursing & Health, 21,* 375–382.

Sandelowski, M. (2000). Whatever happened to qualitative description? *Research in Nursing & Health, 23,* 334–340.

Sandelowski, M. (2001). Real qualitative researchers do not count: The use of numbers in qualitative research. *Research in Nursing & Health, 24*(3), 230–240.

Sandelowski, M. (2002). Reembodying qualitative inquiry. *Qualitative Health Research, 12*(1), 104–115.

Sandelowski, M. (2004a). Counting cats in Zanzibar. *Research in Nursing & Health, 27,* 215–216.

Sandelowski, M. (2004b). Using qualitative research. *Qualitative Health Research, 14*(10), 1366–1386.

Sandelowski, M. (2006). "Meta-Jeopardy": The crisis of representation in qualitative metasynthesis. *Nursing Outlook, 54,* 10–16.

Sandelowski, M., & Barroso, J. (2002). Finding the findings in qualitative studies. *Journal of Nursing Scholarship, 34,* 213–219.

Sandelowski, M., & Barroso, J. (2003a). Classifying the findings in qualitative research. *Qualitative Health Research, 13*(7), 905–923.

Sandelowski, M., & Barroso, J. (2003b). Creating metasummaries of qualitative findings. *Nursing Research, 52,* 226–233.

Sandelowski, M., & Barroso, J. (2003c). Writing the proposal for a qualitative research methodology project. *Qualitative Health Research, 13*(6), 781–820.

Sandelowski, M., & Barroso, J. (2007). *Handbook for synthesizing qualitative research.* New York: Springer.

Sandelowski, M., Davis, D. H., & Harris, B. G. (1989). Artful design: Writing the proposal for research in the naturalist paradigm. *Research in Nursing & Health, 12,* 77–84.

Sandelowski, M., Docherty, S., & Emden, C. (1997b). Qualitative metasynthesis: Issues and techniques. *Research in Nursing & Health, 20,* 365–371.

Sandelowski, M., Trimble, F., Woodard, E. K., & Barroso, J. (2006). From synthesis to script: Transforming qualitative research findings for use in practice. *Qualitative Health Research, 16*(10), 1350–1370.

Sandelowski, M., Voils, C. I., & Barroso, J. (2007). Comparability work and the management of difference in research synthesis studies. *Social Science & Medicine, 64*(236–247).

Sanders, S. (2005). Clever searching for evidence (editorial). *British Medical Journal, 330,* 1162–1163.

Scambler, G., & Hopkins, A. (1990). Generating a model of epileptic stigma: The role of qualitative analysis. *Social Science & Medicine, 30,* 1187–1194.

Schatzman, L., & Strauss, A. L. (1973). *Field research: Strategies for a natural sociology.* Englewood Cliffs, NJ: Prentice–Hall.

Schein, E. H. (1987). *The clinical perspective in fieldwork.* Newbury Park, CA: Sage.

Schneider, J. W., & Conrad, P. (1980). In the closet with illness: Epilepsy, stigma potential and information control. *Social Problems, 28,* 32–44.

Schultz, P. R., & Meleis, A. I. (1988). Nursing epistemology: Traditions, insights, questions. *Image: The Journal of Nursing Scholarship, 20,* 217–221.

Schutz, A. (1932/1967). *The phenomenology of the everyday world* (G. Walsh & F. Lehnert, Trans.). Evanstown, IL: Northwestern University Press.

Schwalbe, M. (1995). The responsibilities of sociological poets. *Qualitative Sociology, 18,* 393–413.

Schwandt, T. A. (1994). Constructivist, interpretivist approaches to human inquiry. In N. K. Denzin & Y. S. Lincoln (Eds.), *Handbook of qualitative research* (pp. 118–137). Thousand Oaks, CA: Sage.

Schwandt, T. A. (1996). Farewell to criteriology. *Qualitative Inquiry, 2,* 58–72.

Schwandt, T. A. (1997). *Qualitative inquiry: A dictionary of terms.* Thousand Oaks, CA: Sage.

Schwartz, H., & Jacobs, J. (1979). *Qualitative sociology: A method to the madness.* New York: Free Press.

Seale, C., & Silverman, D. (1997). Ensuring rigour in qualitative research. *European Journal of Public Health, 7*(4), 379–384.

Sherwood, G. (1999). Meta-synthesis: Merging qualitative studies to develop nursing knowledge. *International Journal for Human Caring, 3*(1), 37–42.

Shusterman, R. (1991). Beneath interpretation. In D. R. Hiley, J. F. Bohman, & R. Shusterman (Eds.), *The interpretive turn: Philosophy, science, culture* (pp. 102-128). Ithaca, NY: Cornell University Press.

Sidani, S., Epstein, D. R., & Moritz, P. (2003). An alternative paradigm for clinical nursing research: An exemplar. *Research in Nursing & Health, 26,* 244-255.

Sieber, J. E. (1993). The ethics and politics of sensitive research. In C. M. Renzetti & R. M. Lee (Eds.), *Researching sensitive topics* (pp. 14-26). Thousand Oaks, CA: Sage.

Sieber, J. E. (1998). Planning ethically responsible research. In L. Bickman & D. J. Rog (Eds.), *Handbook of applied social research methods* (pp. 127-156). Thousand Oaks, CA: Sage.

Silverman, D. (1985). *Qualitative methodology and sociology.* Aldershot, UK: Gower.

Silverman, D. (1993). *Interpreting qualitative data: Methods for analysing talk, text and interaction.* London: Sage.

Silverman, D. (1998). The quality of qualitative health research: The open-ended interview and its alternatives. *Social Sciences in Health, 4*(2), 104-118.

Simmons, S. (1995). From paradigm to method in interpretive action research. *Journal of Advanced Nursing, 21,* 837-844.

Spradley, J. P. (1979). *The ethnographic interview.* New York: Holt, Rinehart & Winston.

Stern, P. N. (1985). Using grounded theory method in nursing research. In M. M. Leininger (Ed.), *Qualitative research methods in nursing* (pp. 149-160). Orlando, FL: Grune & Stratton.

Stern, P. N. (1994). Eroding grounded theory. In J. M. Morse (Ed.), *Critical issues in qualitative research methods* (pp. 212-223). Thousand Oaks, CA: Sage.

Stewart, D. W., & Shamdasani, P. N. (1998). Focus group research: Exploration and discovery. In L. Bickman & D. J. Rog (Eds.), *Handbook of applied social research methods* (pp. 505-526). Thousand Oaks, CA: Sage.

Strauss, A. (1995). Notes on the nature and development of general theories. *Qualitative Inquiry, 1*(1), 7-18.

Strauss, A. L. (1975). *Chronic illness and the quality of life.* St. Louis: Mosby.

Strauss, A. L. (1987). *Qualitative analysis for social scientists.* Cambridge: Cambridge University Press.

Strauss, A. L., & Corbin, J. (1998). *Basics of qualitative research: Grounded theory procedures and techniques* (2nd ed.). Newbury Park, CA: Sage.

Sudnow, D. (1967). *Passing on: The social organization of dying.* Englewood Cliffs, N.J: Prentice-Hall.

Tarlier, D. (2005). Mediating the meaning of evidence through epistemological diversity. *Nursing Inquiry, 12*(2), 126-134.

Thompson, J. L. (1985). Practical discourse in nursing: Going beyond empiricism and historicism. *Advances in Nursing Science, 7*(4), 56-68.

Thorne, S. (1993). *Negotiating health care: The social context of chronic illness.* Newbury Park, CA: Sage.

Thorne, S. (1994). Secondary analysis in qualitative research: Issues and implications. In J. M. Morse (Ed.), *Critical issues in qualitative research methods* (pp. 263–279). Thousand Oaks, CA: Sage.

Thorne, S. (1997). The art (and science) of critiquing qualitative research. In J. M. Morse (Ed.), *Completing a qualitative project: Details and dialogue* (pp. 117–132). Thousand Oaks, CA: Sage.

Thorne, S. (2000a). Data analysis in qualitative rescarch. *Evidence Based Nursing, 3*, 68–70.

Thorne, S. (2000b). Happenings: Off the shelves and into the streets (commentary). *Canadian Journal of Nursing Research, 32*(3), 103–107.

Thorne, S., & Darbyshire, P. (2005). Landmines in the field: A modest proposal for improving the craft of qualitative health research. *Qualitative Health Research, 15*, 1105–1113.

Thorne, S., Jensen, L. A., Kearney, M. H., Noblit, G., & Sandelowski, M. (2004). Reflections on the methodological and ideological agenda in qualitative meta-synthesis. *Qualitative Health Research, 14*, 1342–1365.

Thorne, S., Joachim, G., Paterson, B., & Canam, C. (2002). *Influence of the research frame on qualitatively derived health science knowledge.* Retrieved Jan 1/03 from http://www.ualberta.ca/~ijqm/.

Thorne, S., Radford, J., & McCormick, J. (1997). The multiple meanings of long term gastrostomy in children with severe disability. *Journal of Pediatric Nursing, 12*(2), 89–99.

Thorne, S., Reimer Kirkham, S., & MacDonald-Emes, J. (1997). Interpretive description: A non-categorical qualitative alternative for developing nursing knowledge. *Research in Nursing & Health, 20*(2), 169–177.

Thorne, S., Reimer Kirkham, S., & O'Flynn-Magee, K. (2004). The analytic challenge in interpretive description. *International Journal of Qualitative Methods, 3(2).* Retrieved April 19/04 from http://www.ualberta.ca/~iiqm/backissues/3_1/html/thorneetal.html.

Thorne, S., & Varcoe, C. (1988). The tyranny of feminist methodology in women's health research. *Heath Care for Women International, 19*, 481–493.

Thorne, S. E. (1991). Methodological orthodoxy in qualitative nursing research: Analysis of the issues. *Qualitative Health Research, 1*(2), 178–199.

Thorne, S. E. (2001). The implications of disciplinary agenda on quality criteria for qualitative research. In J. M. Morse, J. Swanson, & A. Kuzel (Eds.), *The nature of qualitative evidence* (pp. 141–159). Thousand Oaks, CA: Sage.

Thorne, S. E., Kazanjian, A., & MacEntee, M. I. (2001). Oral health in long-term care: The implications of organizational culture. *Journal of Aging Studies, 15*, 271–283.

Thorne, S. E., & Paterson, B. L. (2000). Two decades of insider research: What we know and don't know about chronic illness experience. *Annual Review of Nursing Research, 18*, 3–25.

Thorne, S. E., & Robinson, C. A. (1989). Guarded alliance: Health care relationships in chronic illness. *Image: The Journal of Nursing Scholarship, 21*(3), 153–157.

Upshur, R. E. G. (2001). The status of qualitative research as evidence. In J. M. Morse, J. M. Swanson, & A. J. Kuzel (Eds.), *The nature of qualitative evidence* (pp. 5–26). Thousand Oaks, CA: Sage.

Van Kaam, A. (1966). Anthropological phenomenology as a mode of existence. In A. V. Kaam (Ed.), *Existential foundations of psychology* (pp. 231–252). Pittsburgh, PA: Duquesne University Press.

Van Kaam, A. (1969). *Existential foundations of psychology.* New York: Doubleday.

Van Maanen, J. (1988). *Tales of the field: On writing ethnography.* Chicago: University of Chicago Press.

Van Manen, M. (1990). *Researching lived experience: Human science for an action sensitive pedagogy.* New York: State University of New York.

Vidich, A. J., & Lyman, S. M. (1994). Qualitative methods: Their history in sociology and anthropology. In N. K. Denzin & Y. S. Lincoln (Eds.), *Handbook of qualitative research* (pp. 23–59). Thousand Oaks, CA: Sage.

Wagner, E. H., Austin, B. T., Davis, C., Hindmarsh, M., Schaefer, J., & Bonomi, A. (2001). Improving chronic illness care: Translating evidence into action. *Health Affairs (Millwood), 20*(6), 64–78.

Watson, J. (1995). Postmodernism and knowledge development in nursing. *Nursing Science Quarterly, 8*(2), 60–64.

Wilson, H. S., & Hutchinson, S. A. (1997). Presenting qualitative research up close: Visual literacy in poster presentations. In J. M. Morse (Ed.), *Completing a qualitative project: Details and dialogue* (pp. 63–85). Thousand Oaks, CA: Sage.

Wolcott, H. F. (1990). *Writing up qualitative research.* Newbury Park, CA: Sage.

Wolcott, H. F. (1994). *Transforming qualitative data: Description, analysis, and interpretation.* Thousand Oaks, CA: Sage.

Wolcott, H. (1992). Posturing in qualitative inquiry. In M. D. L. Compte, W. L. Millroy, & J. Preissle (Eds.), *The handbook of qualitative research in education* (pp. 3–52). New York: Academic Press.

Yegdich, T. (2000). In the name of Husserl: Nursing in pursuit of the things-in-themselves. *Nursing Inquiry, 7*(1), 29–40.

Sally Thorne, RN, PhD, is Professor and Director of the School of Nursing at the University of British Columbia, in Vancouver, Canada. Her research emphasis for the past 25 years has been the human experience of chronic illness and cancer. Following the initial publication of her methodological work on interpretive description in 1997, she has continued to develop it as a qualitative research approach particularly suited to the research questions generated from within the applied disciplines, including the health professions. Within her program of multidisciplinary team research, she has used interpretive description to advance an understanding of a range of complex and interrelated health issues and to interpret consumer perspectives as a basis from which to strategically reconsider structural and ideological aspects of our health care delivery systems. The interpretive description method has been recognized as a reasoned and accessible approach to generating knowledge that informs practice, attracting an enthusiastic following across the health and other applied disciplines. Dr. Thorne is a widely published author, sought after as a consultant on qualitative methodological issues, and a committed educator. She maintains active service involvements within the professional practice and education sectors, drawing inspiration from human health experience research to bridge the theoretical enterprise with social action and policy processes. Within this context, she has been a champion for the application of qualitative research methodologies to addressing complex health and health care problems, engaging a philosophical analysis of the nature of knowledge claims into considerations of evidence based health care decision making.

INDEX